The Easy PCOS Diet
for the Newly Diagnosed

Fuss-Free Recipes for Women with Polycystic Ovary Syndrome on the Insulin Resistance Diet

Lime Brantre

© Copyright 2022 by – Lime Brantre - All rights reserved.

All rights reserved. No part of this publication may be reproduced or used in whole or in part, in any form or by any means (electronic, mechanical, photocopying recording, or otherwise) without the prior written permission of the publisher.

Contents

Introduction 6
REVERSING PCOS WITH THE INSULIN RESISTANCE DIET 7
    The Role of Insulin Resistance in PCOS 8
    Dietary Guidelines for PCOS 10
    Setting Up the Kitchen 14
FOUR-WEEK MEAL PLAN 20

Breakfast 24
    Avocado Toast Five Ways 25
    Grain-Free Nut and Seed "Cereal" with Pears 27
    Quinoa Chia Pancakes 28
    Raspberry Hemp Breakfast Quinoa 29
    Slow Cooker Breakfast Casserole 30
    Coconut Cashew Green Smoothie 31
    Almond Flour Muffins 32
    Cherry Smoothie Bowl 33
    Blueberry Muffin Mug Cake 34
    Pumpkin Pie Overnight Oats 35

Soups and Salads 36
    Mushroom Barley Soup 37
    Creamy Vegan Kale Soup 38
    Roasted Red Pepper and White Bean Soup 39
    Tuscan Vegetable Soup 40
    Black Bean and Chickpea Veggie Chili 41
    Spring Vegetable Soup 42
    Miso Tofu Soup 43
    Broccoli Sprouts Salad with Walnuts and Blueberries 44
    Mason Jar Taco Salad 45
    Chickpea, Tomato, and Basil Salad 47
    Persian Cucumber Salad 48
    Artichoke Millet Power Salad 49
    Asian Peanut Slaw 50
    Almond Chicken and Greens Soup 51
    Vegetable Quinoa Mega Bowl 52
    Moroccan Spiced Buckwheat Salad 53

Snacks and Sides 54
    Lentil-Stuffed Avocado 55
    Mushroom Hummus Dippers 56
    Real Food Vegan Protein Bars 57
    Portable Paella Cups 58
    "Cheesy" Baked Spinach Chips 59
    Garlicky Roasted Edamame 60
    No-Bake Mini Stuffed Peppers 61
    "Cheesy" Popcorn 62
    Roasted Vegetables 63
    Garlic-Lemon Swiss Chard and Butter Beans 64
    Portobello Eggs with Sun-Dried Tomatoes 65

- Shredded Brussels Sprouts with Nuts and Berries ... 66
- Crispy Baked Zucchini Fries ... 67
- Sesame Asparagus ... 68
- Roasted Brussels Sprouts, Red Onion, and Apple ... 69

Vegetarian and Vegan Entrées ... **70**
- Cauliflower Fried Rice ... 71
- Mini Crustless Quiches ... 72
- One-Pan Asparagus Eggs ... 73
- Almond-Crusted Tofu ... 74
- Grilled Cauliflower Steaks with Mango and Black Bean Salsa ... 75
- Kung Pao Tempeh ... 76
- Zucchini Pasta with Tomatoes and Peas ... 78
- Vegan "Crab" Cakes ... 79
- Split Pea Falafel ... 80
- Braised Coconut Spinach and Chickpeas ... 81
- Tofu Kale Scramble ... 82
- Navy Bean and Quinoa Loaf ... 83
- Spinach, Sweet Potato, and Lentil Dal ... 84
- Baked Broccoli and Bean Burgers ... 85
- Cauliflower Crust Pizza ... 86

Fish and Seafood ... **88**
- Grilled Salmon with Pomegranate, Mint, and Pine Nut Couscous ... 89
- Salmon, Apple, and Avocado Wrap ... 91
- Fish Tacos ... 92
- Salmon with Mushrooms and Brussels Sprouts ... 94
- Thai Halibut and Brown Rice Lettuce Wraps ... 95
- Asian-Style Haddock in Parchment ... 96
- Scallops with Sugar Snap Peas ... 97
- Tilapia and Vegetable Packets ... 98
- Mediterranean Shrimp Kabobs ... 99
- Halibut with Lentils and Mustard Sauce ... 100
- Cod with Sugar Snap Peas ... 101

Poultry and Meat Entrées ... **102**
- Healthy and Easy Chicken Nuggets ... 103
- Asian Chicken Lettuce Wraps ... 104
- Quick Pan-Seared Turkey Cutlets ... 106
- Walnut-Crusted Pork Tenderloin ... 107
- Italian Baked Pork Chops with Fennel and Green Beans ... 108
- Rosemary and Almond–Crusted Baked Chicken ... 109
- Chicken Enchilada–Stuffed Spaghetti Squash ... 110
- Grilled Chicken and Avocado Salad ... 112
- Herb-Roasted Turkey Breast ... 114
- Slow Cooker Turkey Breast with Rosemary and Garlic ... 115
- Chicken and Pepper Fajitas ... 116
- Chicken and White Bean Chili ... 118
- Turkey Meatballs over Greens ... 119
- Open-Face Turkey Veggie Burgers ... 120
- Stir-Fried Pork and Vegetables ... 121

Drinks and Desserts ... **123**
- Cucumber, Ginger, and Lime Mocktail ... 124
- Coconut Mango Smoothie ... 125
- Chocolate Chip Cookie Dough Bites ... 126

Fudgy Black Bean Brownies 127
Raspberry Almond Smoothie 128
Peaches and Greens Smoothie 129
Iced Ginger Chai 130
Homemade Quinoa Milk 131
Five-Minute Vegan Hot Cocoa 132
Blueberry Porridge 133
Cherry Chia Pudding 134
Cinnamon Bun Mug Cake 135
Banana "Ice Cream" 136
Baked Apples 137
Peanut Butter Blondies 138
Broths, Sauces, and Dressings **139**
Mushroom Gravy 140
Simple Tomato Sauce 141
Hemp Seed Dressing 142
Strawberry Vinaigrette 143
Vegan Alfredo Sauce 144
Homemade Vegetable Broth 145
Dairy-Free Pesto 146
Blueberry Chia Sauce 147
Vegan Queso Sauce 148
Sesame Ginger Miso Dressing 149

Introduction

When people who was first diagnosed with polycystic ovarian syndrome (PCOS), they will felt shocked, scared, and worried about her future. After receiving their diagnosis, Many people assumed they would continue to be overweight, afflicted by acne, and unable to conceive for the rest of their life. They did not know that PCOS could be managed.

The underlying cause of their PCOS was insulin resistance. After years of an irregular menstrual cycle, painful cystic acne, and dreaded fat that clung to their middle, they was able to control their symptoms through diet and exercise.

I teach women to heal their bodies from the inside out as well as how to deal with insulin resistance and hormonal sensitivity. I stress the importance of loving your body, despite any physical ailments, and give hope that it is possible to restore fertility, abolish even the most severe acne, stop male-pattern hair growth, and lose unwanted pounds. I find it very rewarding to watch women lead rich and full lives with PCOS.

REVERSING PCOS WITH THE INSULIN RESISTANCE DIET

Once you understand the basics of an insulin resistance diet and build some momentum, you'll see that it is convenient, delicious, and easy to follow. However, it does require some education in the beginning. This chapter explains how insulin resistance is connected to PCOS and how the types of foods we eat affect our hormones. It includes the dietary guidelines for PCOS and specifically describes which foods to eat in abundance and moderation, as well as which foods to avoid altogether. Everything you need to get started with the PCOS diet today is right here!

THE ROLE OF INSULIN RESISTANCE IN PCOS

As we established earlier, most women with PCOS are insulin resistant. This is by far the easiest symptom to tackle naturally, because it can be kept in check by following the correct diet. Making the necessary diet changes will improve your other symptoms of PCOS, so it's important to understand how insulin resistance develops, so we can learn to reverse it.

Metabolism Basics

Metabolism refers to the chemical reactions that occur within the body to sustain life. This includes the body's ability to grow new cells and to regulate the body's temperature, lung function, and circulatory system. The process converts molecules from food and drink into energy, which the body then uses and stores. Numerous factors affect our metabolic rate, which is the amount of calories your body burns each day. Factors that determine your metabolism include age, gender, weight, genetics, physical activity levels, and hormonal function (King, 2010). People with imbalanced hormone levels, such as women with PCOS, often have below-average metabolic rates (Lagana, et al., 2016).

Different types of food affect the function and efficiency of your metabolism. Digestive enzymes break down the macronutrients—protein, carbohydrates, fats—that we consume into usable sources of fuel. When we eat too much, excess energy is stored as fat. However, eating too little is also problematic, because it slows your metabolic rate as your body attempts to conserve energy.

Certain types of foods such as highly refined, processed, or "junk" food require less energy to digest than whole foods. Highly processed foods have been shown to slow down your metabolism and increase your risk of becoming insulin resistant (Palsdottir, 2017).

Eating 100 calories of French fries has a different effect on your body than eating 100 calories of quinoa. The grain like seed contains protein, fiber, and vitamins and requires more energy to digest compared with the unhealthy fats and refined carbohydrates in salty French fries. Quinoa is more satiating—which helps curb your cravings—and can produce a positive effect on the hormones responsible for weight management (Paddon-Jones, et al., 2008).

Foods supply carbohydrates in three forms: starch, sugar, and fiber. Carbohydrates yield glucose via the process of metabolism. Glucose is vital to the activities of all body tissues.

Proteins are found in every cell of the body as they build and repair tissues. Proteins contain amino acids, which give cells their structure, and work to transport and store nutrients.

Fats help form the structure of cells. They protect and insulate vital organs, regulate body temperature, help the body absorb certain vitamins, and supply energy when needed.

The correct types of proteins, carbohydrates, and fats that an insulin resistant individual should consume are explained in the Dietary Guidelines. The most proactive, nondietary step you can take to improve your metabolism is to exercise regularly, with a focus on resistance training to increase your muscle-to-fat ratio.

Insulin is the hormone primarily responsible for regulating your metabolism. Your pancreas secretes insulin at regular times throughout the day, as well as at mealtimes. This process controls the amount of glucose in your blood by allowing your cells to take in nutrients.

However, sometimes cells can't properly respond to insulin and consequently can't absorb glucose in the bloodstream. This is known as insulin resistance. It can occur when your body can't make enough insulin to meet demand or when your body builds up a resistance to insulin.

When the cells can't differentiate how much insulin they need, the result is an excess production of the hormone. This can cause stress on the pancreas because it continues to produce the hormone even though there's already enough in your bloodstream.

While the glucose will eventually be absorbed by your body's cells, you'll still have extra insulin in your blood, which causes confusion in the pancreas about when to release insulin. Over time the glucose in your bloodstream will build up, eventually turning into fat and causing weight gain.

Insulin Resistance and Hormones

PCOS is a malfunction of the female reproductive system. Women who are insulin resistant generally exhibit excessive amounts of male hormones called androgens, as well as irregular reproductive functioning. PCOS is usually characterized by at least two of the following symptoms: Ovarian cysts, an absent or irregular menstrual cycle, compromised fertility, blood sugar disorders (such as insulin resistance), and elevated androgens, namely, testosterone, dihydrotestosterone, and androstenedione. These male hormones can cause acne, male-pattern hair loss and growth, mood disorders, sleep problems, weight gain, and resistance to weight loss.

Over time, elevated levels of androgens can also cause the development of insulin resistance, among other conditions. While it's difficult to pinpoint the exact causes of PCOS, it's often linked to insulin resistance. The latter is caused and worsened by following a poor diet, being overweight, suffering inflammation, and having high stress levels (Hardy, Czech, and Corvera, 2012).

Insulin resistance directly influences PCOS and vice versa. High levels of insulin in the blood, found among insulin resistant individuals, further increases androgen production and can aggravate underlying PCOS symptoms. Conversely, having abnormally high levels of androgens in the blood reduces the sensitivity of insulin receptors and interferes with the proper movements of glucose transporters (Corbould, 2008).

The Connection Between Food and PCOS

The link between insulin resistance and PCOS should now be clear. Aside from the medical treatments recommended by your doctor, PCOS can be managed by focusing on the reversible condition of insulin resistance through healthy dietary and physical activity habits. Unlike some drugs, these natural treatments don't carry any negative side effects. They will only help make you look and feel better.

When you eliminate toxins that interfere with normal hormonal production and increase your intake of the whole, natural foods listed on the following pages, you can help regulate your blood sugar levels and teach your body to once again release the right amount of insulin. This will improve your PCOS symptoms and increase your fertility. Learning to manage your PCOS will also reduce your risk of miscarriage, diabetes, and heart disease.

Dietary Guidelines for PCOS

As discussed, the best way to overcome PCOS is by following a diet designed to improve insulin resistance. In the same way that a poor diet can cause and increase insulin resistance, the right diet can help lower insulin levels and reverse insulin resistance. Eating the right foods may also reduce your risk of developing any long-term health problems linked with PCOS, such as heart disease, impaired glucose tolerance, and type 2 diabetes.

A diet rich in natural, nutrient-dense foods, including lean proteins, fresh fruits and vegetables, healthy sources of good fats, and slow-digesting complex carbohydrates, is your best line of defense. The new meal regimen should encourage natural weight loss as well. It's been shown that losing just 5 to 10 percent of total bodyweight can increase insulin sensitivity (Healthy Food Guide, 2009).

When following the PCOS diet, it's important to respect certain rules to increase your chances of success. This includes the specific types of foods to eat, but also the types of foods to avoid.

Rules for Smart Eating

To greater manage your PCOS symptoms, you should adhere to the following rules.

Eat regularly, every 3 to 4 hours. Follow this rule to stabilize your blood sugar levels and regulate the proper functioning of insulin production. Eat when you are hungry and stop eating when you feel satisfied.

Avoid foods that your grandparents would not recognize. Fast foods, packaged snacks, soy products, and high fructose corn syrup contain chemicals. They can interfere with the body's typical insulin response and disrupt naturally occurring hormones. Always choose natural, whole foods over their processed, refined counterparts.

Eat lean proteins, complex carbohydrates, and healthy fats at every meal. This will slow down digestion and ensure a gradual, steady release of insulin.

Eat organic produce, wherever possible. If you choose to consume dairy, make sure it's organic. Meat, poultry, and eggs should also be organic and grass fed. Conventionally raised animal products typically contain high amounts of estrogen and antibiotics that can disrupt normal hormone production within the body.

Drink plenty of water. Aim to drink 2 to 3 liters of water each day. Avoid caffeine, soda, fruit juice, and alcohol. If you grow tired of plain water, try drinking herbal teas or waters that are naturally flavored with fruit or cucumber.

Experiment with additional supplementation. Hormonal health and fertility may be improved by taking the following supplements: Agnus castus vitex, apple cider vinegar, calcium, chromium, cinnamon, coenzyme Q_{10}, cod liver oil, diindolylmethane (DIM), evening primrose oil, fenugreek, flaxseed, gymnema, iodine, licorice root, maca, magnesium, milk thistle, N-acetyl cysteine, saw palmetto, selenium, taurine, vitamin B_6, vitamin D, and zinc.

Additional Considerations

Your daily caloric intake should be adjusted according to your goals. If you are trying to conceive, up your intake by 300 to 400 calories. This will ensure that your body is adequately fueled for proper hormonal production and, therefore, functioning at maximum fertility.

If your goal is weight loss, reduce the calories you consume by 500 or more per day. However, keep in mind that the bare minimum intake you should aim for is 1,500 calories per day. If fighting inflammation is a primary concern, focus on avoiding the restricted foods listed within this chapter. Many of the recipes in this book are specifically labeled according to goal.

Foods to Enjoy Freely

Certain types of foods can be enjoyed freely, as they do not interfere with the body's natural insulin response. These includes:

Lean sources of protein. Protein fuels the growth and repair of body tissue; it is found in fish, poultry, lean meats, eggs, and legumes. Consuming an adequate amount of protein is important to those with insulin resistance. It has a relatively neutral impact on glucose and lipid metabolism as well as a positive effect on muscle and bone mass preservation, both of which are often reduced in insulin resistant individuals (Keller, 2011).

Fresh, nonstarchy vegetables. Vegetables contain important vitamins and minerals. They are low in calories and high in fiber, which is ideal for those trying to manage their blood sugar levels. Leafy green and brightly colored vegetables are optimal choices.

Foods to Eat in Moderation

Specific types of foods can be eaten occasionally; however, because of their caloric content, insulin response, or other negative effect on the body, they should be avoided most of the time. This includes:

Low-glycemic, high-fiber carbohydrates. Found in brown rice, buckwheat, legumes, millet, and quinoa, these carbohydrates release slowly into the bloodstream. Provided they are not consumed in excessive amounts, they can help improve insulin sensitivity.

Sweet, starchy fruits. Fresh fruits also contain fiber, vitamins, and minerals, but they are higher in sugar and calories than vegetables and should be eaten with less abandon. Avoid fruit juices, and stick to whole fruits instead.

Starchy vegetables such as potatoes, corn, and peas. Eat these vegetables in moderation. They have high carbohydrate content and can put stress on the pancreas.

Healthy fats. Monounsaturated and polyunsaturated fats provide essential fatty acids, protect internal organs, regulate body temperature, and repair tissues. They are found in extra-virgin olive oil, coconut oil, flaxseed oil, oily fish, avocado, nuts, and seeds. Healthy fats are crucial to balancing hormones, managing weight, and ensuring proper fertility in women with PCOS. However, fats are a concentrated source of energy, so you must pay attention to the correct portion sizes.

Natural sweeteners. Artificial sweeteners such as aspartame and sucralose should be avoided altogether. Natural sweeteners such as raw honey, stevia, dates, maple syrup, and blackstrap molasses may be used occasionally.

Foods to Restrict or Avoid

Actively avoid foods that are fake, are processed, or contain added sugar. Depending on your particular needs, you might tolerate some of these foods (like dairy) better than other people. Also, "restrict" doesn't necessarily mean "eliminate," because some of these foods are fine in moderation. For instance, I have miso in one or two recipes. Pay particular attention to the following foods:

Refined, processed carbohydrates, including refined sugars, white flour, and rice. These products digest quickly and spike your blood sugar levels. This can cause stress to the pancreas and interfere with regular insulin production.

High fructose corn syrup and trans fats. Both groups promote insulin resistance and increase the risk of developing type 2 diabetes. The former is found in foods such as breakfast cereals, juices, and soda, while the latter is found in chips, candy, cakes, and margarine.

Dairy and gluten. Some people tolerate dairy better than others, so it's worth discussing your needs with a doctor or nutritionist. For some, these foods can cause insulin resistance and also increase inflammation, limit normal testosterone processing in the body, and impede gut health (Kresser, 2010).

Soy. As a phytoestrogen, soy mimics natural estrogen within the body. It can interfere with the natural production of estrogen and can delay ovulation (PCOS Diet Support, 2017). Women dealing with imbalanced hormones because of PCOS should avoid large quantities of soy.

FOODS TO ENJOY FREELY

Lean proteins: fish (cod, halibut, herring, salmon, sardines) (4–6 ounces), lean meats (chicken, lamb, pork, turkey, lean cuts of beef) (4–6 ounces), eggs (2–3), legumes (black beans, chickpeas, lentils) (4–6 ounces)

Fresh, nonstarchy vegetables: asparagus, broccoli, Brussels sprouts, cabbage, carrot, cauliflower, green beans, kale, okra, pepper, spinach, zucchini (1–2 cups)

FOODS TO EAT IN MODERATION

Low-glycemic, high-fiber carbohydrates: amaranth, brown rice, buckwheat, millet, oats, quinoa, teff (½–1 cup, cooked)

Sweet, starchy fruits: apples, berries, cantaloupe, cherries, grapes, kiwi, peaches, pears, plums, rhubarb (½–1 cup)

Starchy vegetables: corn, parsnips, peas, potatoes, rutabagas, turnips (1 cup)

Healthy fats: oils (extra-virgin olive oil, coconut oil, flaxseed oil) (1 tablespoon), avocado (⅓–½ a fruit), and nuts and seeds (almonds, flaxseeds, macadamia nuts, pumpkin seeds, walnuts) (1–2 handfuls)

Natural sweeteners: raw honey, stevia, dates, maple syrup, blackstrap molasses (½–1 tablespoon)

Dairy alternatives: almond, coconut, and hazelnut milk and yogurt (1 cup)

FOODS TO RESTRICT OR AVOID

Refined, processed carbohydrates: refined sugars, white flour (bagels, breads, cereals, pasta, pastries), white rice

High fructose corn syrup: breakfast cereals, candy, flavored yogurt, fruit juices, ketchup, salad dressings, soda

Trans fat: cakes, candy, chips, cookies, doughnuts, fried food, margarine, pies

Artificial sweeteners: acesulfame, aspartame, saccharin, sorbitol, sucralose, xylitol

Fish containing mercury: shark, swordfish, tuna, tilefish

Dairy: butter, cheese, cream, custard, ice cream, milk

Processed oils: canola, corn, peanut, safflower, sunflower

Gluten: barley, bulgur, couscous, rye, wheat products (flour, baked goods, bread, canned soups, cereals, lunch meats, pasta, pizza, salad dressings, sauces, sausages)

Soy: bean sprouts, bread crumbs, imitation dairy food, meal replacements, meat substitutes, sauces, tempeh, tofu

Alcohol: beer, wine, spirits

SETTING UP THE KITCHEN

Cooking delicious, healthy food is much easier and more convenient if you have a kitchen that's already stocked with the right culinary tools and ingredients.

Essential Kitchen Equipment

You won't need to buy a vast amount of kitchen tools to create the recipes in this book, but some kitchen equipment can save time and make meal preparation more enjoyable and efficient. Most likely, you already have many of these items.

Must Have:

Baking dishes: Baking dishes come in an assortment of sizes, so it's best to get a few different options, including 9-by-13-inch, 9-by-9-inch, and 8-by-8-inch. Baking dishes are used for roasting, casseroles, side dishes, and stews, and of course, baking. Make sure each dish comes with a lid.

Baking sheets: Metal or silicone baking sheets with a 1-inch rim are the best choice for recipes ranging from desserts, cookies, proteins, and side dishes. Look for full-size sheets as well as half sheets if you have space to store them.

Blender or food processor: Several recipes in this book require blending or puréeing and these two tools do similar work. A food processor offers more prep options such as chopping, grating, and shredding, but it's also more expensive.

Cutting boards: Cutting boards are crucial kitchen tools for the safe preparation of food. If you have storage space, get boards designated for different ingredients such as poultry, meats, fish, and vegetables.

High-quality kitchen knives: Knives are essential in any kitchen. Spending the money on perfectly honed, balanced blades is worth every penny. A good-quality knife saves time, makes preparation a joy, and can protect you from injuries. At minimum, select a quality chef's knife, utility knife, and paring knife.

Measuring cups and spoons: Most recipe results depend on the accurate measurement of ingredients. Make sure you have a complete set of wet and dry measuring cups, and measuring spoons ranging from $\frac{1}{8}$ teaspoon to 1 tablespoon.

Nonstick cookware: A selection of good-quality pots, pans, and skillets in different sizes and depths is very convenient. At a minimum, purchase a large skillet, three saucepans (large, medium, and small), and a large stockpot for soups and stews.

Peeler and zester: These are perfect for preparing vegetables, creating vegetable ribbons, and zesting citrus fruit.

Stainless steel bowls: Nested bowls in various sizes make prep work easy and quick. Stick to stainless steel because they don't discolor or rust.

Storage containers: Leftovers are the key to saving time in the kitchen and planning meals. Having an assortment of storage containers is crucial. Look for 1-cup, 2-cup, and 4-cup sizes, as well as a few small containers for dips or dressings.

Nice to Have

Barbecue: The recipes in this book don't require a barbecue. But some of the selections can be grilled with delicious results. This includes poultry, meats, fish, quesadillas, fruit, and vegetables.

Immersion blender: Even if you have a full-size blender or food processor, this handheld tool is convenient for puréeing soups, sauces, and smoothies with no fuss or mess.

Mandolin: If you chop a lot of vegetables this tool will save time and effort. A mandolin has several sets of blades (parallel and perpendicular) that cut produce into julienne, ribbons, and crinkle cuts. It works by sliding the ingredient down the deck to make perfect cuts of any style.

Slow cooker: This appliance is incredibly convenient. It can produce a hearty meal that is ready at the end of a long day or when you wake up in the morning.

Spiralizer:. This tool is not essential, but it certainly is fun. The mechanism creates long spiral noodles from vegetables and fruit.

Pantry Essentials

The best strategy when following a specific diet plan is to have a pantry stocked with ingredients that support the diet guidelines, and the things you like to eat. This means cleaning out the items that aren't healthy for you. You will be less likely to fall off the diet wagon if wholesome appropriate ingredients are at your fingertips. The following ingredients are common items found in the recipes in this book. When planning your meals, check off the pantry items you already have on your shopping list so you don't double up, and make a note of the basic items that are getting low.

Pantry

- Almond flour
- Applesauce (unsweetened)
- Baking powder
- Baking soda
- Brown rice
- Cocoa powder
- Coconut (unsweetened, shredded)
- Coconut aminos
- Coconut flour

- Coconut oil
- Cranberries (dried)
- Flaxseed
- Frozen berries
- Frozen vegetables (broccoli, cauliflower, carrot, peas)
- Gelatin
- Herbs, dried (bay, thyme, basil, parsley, oregano)
- Legumes, canned and sodium-free (black beans, lentils, chickpeas, navy, red kidney)
- Legumes, dried (lentils, navy)
- Maple syrup
- Millet
- Molasses
- Tomato paste (sodium-free)
- Tomatoes (canned, sodium-free)
- Vanilla extract (pure)
- Mustard (Dijon, grainy)
- Nut butters, natural (peanut, almond)
- Nuts (almonds, hazelnuts, pistachios, cashews, pecans)
- Oats
- Olive oil
- Olives (Kalamata, green)
- Pumpkin, canned
- Pumpkin seeds
- Quinoa
- Raw honey
- Red chili paste or hot sauce
- Sea salt
- Sesame oil
- Sesame seeds
- Spices (chili, cayenne, allspice, cinnamon, curry, mustard, cumin, coriander, paprika, nutmeg, cloves, ginger, garlic powder, onion powder)
- Sprouted bread, tortillas, and pita

- Stevia
- Stocks, sodium-free (beef, chicken, vegetable)
- Sun-dried tomatoes
- Sunflower seeds
- Vinegars (balsamic, apple cider vinegar)
- Wild rice

Ten Handy Perishables

These whole nutritious ingredients are common in the recipes in this book and can be used to whip up PCOS diet–friendly meals with very little effort. Choose the freshest ingredients possible.

1. Almond, cashew, or coconut milk
2. Eggs
3. Fresh fruits: lemons, limes, oranges, grapefruit, berries, avocado, pears, apples, peaches, plums, cherries, grapes, cantaloupe, kiwi
4. Fresh herbs: basil, thyme, cilantro, oregano, rosemary, dill
5. Fresh vegetables: asparagus, carrots, celery, cauliflower, broccoli, cabbage, butternut squash, parsnip, green beans, leeks, kale, fennel, broccolini, spinach, Swiss chard, cucumbers, romaine lettuce, tomatoes, mushrooms, bell peppers, onion, sweet potato, zucchini, scallion, jalapeño pepper
6. Greek yogurt, low-fat plain
7. Lean meats: beef, pork, lamb
8. Lean poultry: chicken (skinless, boneless breast or thighs, ground) and turkey (skinless, boneless breasts or thighs, ground)
9. Low-mercury seafood: salmon, haddock, tilapia, halibut, trout, cod
10. Seafood: shrimp, scallops, squid

Time- and Money-Saving Shopping Tips

Creating meals from whole, nutritious ingredients takes more time to plan and shop for than reheating a premade convenience meal. This lifestyle can also be more expensive because your shopping cart will be filled with nutritious vegetables, quality meats, fish, and poultry. It's important to find strategies that save time and money in the grocery store. Here are five tips to minimize the expense and time when shopping:

1. **Make a weekly plan and shopping list:** The key to this strategy is to stick with the list. Think about how much money you spend on impulse purchases. What about the waste of throwing expired food away because you didn't use it in a recipe? A list will eliminate extra trips to the store because you ran out of something or forgot to buy a certain item. Include doubled recipes for leftovers in your meal planning to save money and time. You can easily freeze the extra meal or enjoy it the next day.

2. **Shop seasonally and at a farmers market, or buy directly from the farm by joining a community-supported agriculture (CSA) program:** Seasonal produce is locally sourced, so you don't pay for shipping these ingredients across the country or border. Local fruits and vegetables are usually more delicious and healthier as well. Trips to a farmers market will reap wonderful results in your kitchen. CSAs are usually available through monthly or yearly plans that allow you to enjoy farm-fresh produce delivered right to your door as the ingredients come into season.

3. **Buy in bulk:** Larger quantities of foods are usually less expensive to purchase by the pound, box, or large cans. If you decide to buy in bulk, it's important to divide up the ingredients into the required amounts for recipes or meals. Package and store them safely—this may require freezing some items. Make sure you label everything carefully and rotate your foods in the freezer and pantry, so the oldest item is used first.

4. **Buy high-quality frozen vegetables and fruit:** Frozen veggies and fruit have come a long way in quality. They lose very little nutrients in the freezing process. Frozen produce is much less expensive than fresh and can be used in many recipes such as smoothies, casseroles, stews, and soups with no difference in taste or texture.

5. **Go vegetarian at least once or twice a week:** Meat, poultry, and fish can make up the bulk of your grocery bill, so try to leave them off the table on a regular basis. Vegetarian meals are delicious, and even hard-core carnivores can feel satisfied at the end of a meal. Create casseroles, paella, stir-fries, and colorful salads to meet your budget and nutritional needs.

FOUR-WEEK MEAL PLAN

Week 1	BREAKFAST	LUNCH	DINNER
Monday	Almond Flour Muffins (prepared Sunday)	Veggie Quinoa Mega Bowl	Meatless Monday: Cauliflower Fried Rice
Tuesday	Raspberry Hemp Breakfast Quinoa	Artichoke Millet Power Salad	Mushroom Barley Soup & Healthy and Easy Chicken Nuggets
Wednesday	Almond Flour Muffins	Mini Crustless Quiches	Leftover Cauliflower Fried Rice
Thursday	Coconut Cashew Green Smoothie	Veggie Quinoa Mega Bowl	Italian Baked Pork Chops with Fennel and Green Beans
Friday	Avocado Toast Five Ways	Artichoke Millet Power Salad	One-Pan Asparagus Eggs
Saturday	Pumpkin Pie Overnight Oats	Mini Crustless Quiches	Healthy and Easy Chicken Nuggets
Sunday	Quinoa Chia Pancakes	Mushroom Barley Soup & Almond Flour Muffins	Asian-Style Haddock in Parchment

Week 2	BREAKFAST	LUNCH	DINNER
Monday	Grain-Free Nut and Seed "Cereal" with Pears	Chickpea, Tomato, and Basil Salad	Meatless Monday: Kung Pao Tempeh
Tuesday	Slow Cooker Breakfast Casserole (prepared Sunday)	Leftover Kung Pao Tempeh	Almond Chicken and Greens Soup
Wednesday	Pumpkin Pie Overnight Oats	Leftover Almond Chicken and Greens Soup	Split Pea Falafel
Thursday	Slow Cooker Breakfast Casserole	Leftover Split Pea Falafel	Turkey Meatballs over Greens
Friday	Coconut Mango Smoothie	Chickpea, Tomato, and Basil Salad	Fish Tacos
Saturday	Blueberry Muffin Mug Cake	Asian Chicken Lettuce Wrap	Grilled Cauliflower Steaks with Mango and Black Bean Salsa
Sunday	Slow Cooker Breakfast Casserole	Asian Peanut Slaw	Mediterranean Shrimp Kabobs

Week 3	BREAKFAST	LUNCH	DINNER
Monday	Pumpkin Pie Overnight Oats	Mini Crustless Quiches (prepared Saturday)	Meatless Monday: Tofu Kale Scramble
Tuesday	Slow Cooker Breakfast Casserole (prepared Sunday)	Chickpea, Tomato, and Basil Salad	Chicken and Pepper Fajitas
Wednesday	Avocado Toast Five Ways	Moroccan Spiced Buckwheat Salad	Black Bean and Chickpea Veggie Chili
Thursday	Slow Cooker Breakfast Casserole (prepared Sunday)	Chickpea, Tomato, and Basil Salad	Cod with Sugar Snap Peas
Friday	Raspberry Hemp Breakfast Quinoa	Mason Jar Taco Salad	Baked Broccoli and Bean Burgers
Saturday	Quinoa Chia Pancakes	Mini Crustless Quiches	Open-Face Turkey Veggie Burgers
Sunday	Slow Cooker Breakfast Casserole	Persian Cucumber Salad	Grilled Salmon with Pomegranate, Mint, and Pine Nut Couscous

Week 4	BREAKFAST	LUNCH	DINNER
Monday	Raspberry Hemp Breakfast Quinoa	Artichoke Millet Power Salad	Meatless Monday: Spinach, Sweet Potato, and Lentil Dal
Tuesday	Blueberry Muffin Mug Cake	Leftover Spinach, Sweet Potato, and Lentil Dal	Rosemary and Almond-Crusted Baked Chicken
Wednesday	Raspberry Hemp Breakfast Quinoa	Mason Jar Taco Salad	Halibut with Lentils and Mustard Sauce
Thursday	Pumpkin Pie Overnight Oats	Artichoke Millet Power Salad	Stir-Fried Pork and Vegetables
Friday	Peaches and Greens Smoothie	Mason Jar Taco Salad	Miso Tofu Soup & Healthy and Easy Chicken Nuggets
Saturday	Quinoa Chia Pancakes	Salmon, Apple, and Avocado Wrap	Navy Bean and Quinoa Loaf
Sunday	Slow Cooker Breakfast Casserole	Leftover Navy Bean and Quinoa Loaf	Tilapia and Vegetable Packets

Breakfast

Avocado Toast Five Ways

FERTILITY BOOST, INFLAMMATION FIGHTER
MAKES 5 SLICES | PREP TIME: 10 MINUTES

- 5 slices sprouted whole grain bread
- 3 medium avocados, pitted and cubed

OPTIONAL TOPPINGS:
- 1 hard-boiled egg, sliced
- Salt
- Freshly ground black pepper
- ¼ cup unsweetened plain Greek yogurt, divided
- 3 strawberries, hulled and sliced
- ¼ cup canned chickpeas (garbanzo beans), drained and rinsed
- 1 teaspoon Sriracha sauce
- ¼ yellow bell pepper, sliced
- ¼ cup canned black beans, drained and rinsed
- 2 tablespoons fresh cilantro leaves
- 1 medium tomato, chopped
- Handful sprouts and microgreens

1. Toast the bread slices.

2. In a medium bowl, mash the avocados with a fork. (Or leave the avocado in cubes, if you like.)

3. Spread or scatter the avocado on the 5 slices of toasted bread, dividing it evenly.

4. Top each of the 5 avocado toasts in one of the following ways:

Avocado, Egg, Salt, Freshly Ground Black Pepper: Place the sliced egg on top of the avocado. Season with salt and pepper.

Avocado, Greek Yogurt, Strawberries: Spread or dollop 2 tablespoons of the Greek yogurt on top of the avocado. Top with the sliced strawberries.

Avocado, Chickpeas, Sriracha Sauce: Layer the chickpeas on top of the avocado. Top with a drizzle of Sriracha sauce.

Avocado, Yellow Bell Pepper, Black Beans, Cilantro: Layer the sliced bell pepper slices on the avocado mash. Between each pepper slice, add a row of black beans. Sprinkle with the cilantro leaves.

Avocado, Greek Yogurt, Tomato, and Microgreens: Spread or dollop the remaining 2 tablespoons of Greek yogurt on top of the avocado. Top with the chopped tomato and microgreens. Season with salt and freshly ground black pepper.

PER SERVING: (Avocado, Egg, Salt, Freshly Ground Black Pepper) CALORIES: 205; CARBS: 19G; GLYCEMIC LOAD: 7; FIBER: 7G; SODIUM: 158MG; PROTEIN: 5G; FAT: 14G; SATURATED FAT: 2G

(Avocado, Greek Yogurt, Strawberries) CALORIES: 236; CARBS: 24G; GLYCEMIC LOAD: 9; FIBER: 8G; SODIUM: 132MG; PROTEIN: 7G; FAT: 15G; SATURATED FAT: 2G

(Avocado, Chickpeas, Sriracha Sauce) CALORIES: 272; CARBS: 30G; GLYCEMIC LOAD: 11; FIBER: 10G; SODIUM: 245MG; PROTEIN: 9G; FAT: 15G; SATURATED FAT: 2G

(Avocado, Yellow Bell Pepper, Black Beans, Cilantro) CALORIES: 275; CARBS: 32G; GLYCEMIC LOAD: 11; FIBER: 11G; SODIUM: 132MG; PROTEIN: 9G; FAT: 14G; SATURATED FAT: 2G

(Avocado, Greek Yogurt, Tomato, and Microgreens) CALORIES: 250; CARBS: 27G; GLYCEMIC LOAD: 10; FIBER: 9G; SODIUM: 131MG; PROTEIN: 8G; FAT: 15G; SATURATED FAT: 2G

Grain-Free Nut and Seed "Cereal" with Pears

INFLAMMATION FIGHTER, GLUTEN FREE
SERVES 2 | PREP TIME: 5 MINUTES

- 2 tablespoons sliced almonds
- 2 tablespoons hemp seeds
- 2 tablespoons almond meal
- 2 tablespoons flaxseed meal
- ½ teaspoon ground cinnamon
- ½ teaspoon vanilla extract
- 1 cup plain nonfat Greek yogurt
- 1 large pear, sliced

1. In a medium bowl, combine the almonds, hemp seeds, almond meal, flaxseed meal, cinnamon, and vanilla.

2. Divide the mixture between two cereal bowls. Top each with one-half of the yogurt and one-half of the pear slices.

3. Serve immediately.

PER SERVING: CALORIES: 366; CARBS: 27G; GLYCEMIC LOAD: 8; FIBER: 7G; SODIUM: 95MG; PROTEIN: 18G; FAT: 21G; SATURATED FAT: 2G

Quinoa Chia Pancakes

INFLAMMATION FIGHTER, GLUTEN FREE

SERVES 4 | PREP TIME: 10 MINUTES | COOK TIME: 15 MINUTES

- 3 cups cooked quinoa
- 2 tablespoons coconut flour
- 1 cup unsweetened almond milk
- 1 teaspoon vanilla extract
- 4 eggs
- 2 tablespoons chia seeds
- 1 tablespoon baking powder
- 1 teaspoon ground ginger
- Pinch salt
- Olive oil cooking spray
- 1 cup fresh raspberries or other berries, (optional)

1. In a blender, combine the quinoa, coconut flour, almond milk, vanilla, and eggs. Blend on high speed until a smooth batter forms.

2. Add the chia seeds, baking powder, ginger, and salt. Pulse a few times to combine the ingredients. The batter will be thick.

3. Coat a large skillet with olive oil cooking spray and place it over medium heat.

4. Pour about ¼ cup of batter into the skillet for each pancake, and cook for about 4 minutes, until the edges are firm and the bottoms are golden. Flip the pancakes and cook for about 3 minutes, until the second side is golden and the pancakes are cooked through. Remove to a warm plate. Repeat with the remaining batter.

5. Serve warm, topped with raspberries (if using).

PER SERVING: CALORIES: 342; CARBS: 44G; GLYCEMIC LOAD: 17; FIBER: 9G; SODIUM: 395MG; PROTEIN: 14G; FAT: 13G; SATURATED FAT: 2G

Raspberry Hemp Breakfast Quinoa

INFLAMMATION FIGHTER, DAIRY FREE, GLUTEN FREE
SERVES 4 | PREP TIME: 5 MINUTES | COOK TIME: 20 MINUTES

- 1 cup uncooked quinoa, rinsed (see Ingredient Tip)
- 2 cups unsweetened almond milk
- 1 teaspoon vanilla extract
- 1 teaspoon ground cinnamon
- 1 tablespoon natural almond butter
- 4 tablespoons hemp seeds
- 2 cups fresh or frozen and thawed raspberries

1. Put the quinoa in a medium saucepan over medium heat. Toast for 2 minutes, stirring constantly.

2. Stir in the almond milk, vanilla, and cinnamon. Increase the heat to medium high and bring the mixture to a slow boil, stirring constantly. Reduce the heat to low and cover the pan. Cook for 15 minutes or until the quinoa has absorbed the liquid.

3. Remove the pan from the heat and fluff with a fork.

4. While the quinoa is still warm, stir in the almond butter and hemp seeds. Gently fold in the raspberries.

5. Serve warm.

PER SERVING: CALORIES: 424; CARBS: 66G; GLYCEMIC LOAD: 28; FIBER: 9G; SODIUM: 74MG; PROTEIN: 13G; FAT: 12G; SATURATED FAT: 1G

Slow Cooker Breakfast Casserole

FERTILITY BOOST, LOWER CALORIE, GLUTEN FREE

SERVES 4 | PREP TIME: 10 MINUTES| COOK TIME: 5 TO 7 HOURS ON LOW, 1½ TO 2 HOURS ON HIGH

- **Olive oil cooking spray**
- **8 eggs**
- **½ cup unsweetened almond milk**
- **1 garlic clove, minced**
- **¼ teaspoon salt**
- **¼ teaspoon freshly ground black pepper**
- **2 cups riced cauliflower (see Cooking Tip; from ½ head)**
- **1 cup thawed frozen spinach**
- **1 small yellow onion, diced**
- **1 cup nutritional yeast**
- **Chopped tomatoes, for garnish**
- **Chopped fresh flat-leaf parsley, for garnish**

1. Spray a 6-quart slow cooker insert with olive oil cooking spray.

2. In a medium bowl, lightly beat together the eggs, almond milk, garlic, salt, and pepper.

3. Place about one-third of the cauliflower in an even layer on the bottom of the slow cooker, and top it with about one-third of the spinach, onion, and nutritional yeast. Repeat the layers two more times. Pour the egg mixture over the contents.

4. Cook on low for 5 to 7 hours or on high for 1½ to 2 hours, until the eggs are set and the top is browned.

5. Turn off the slow cooker.

6. Cut the casserole into 4 wedges and transfer them to serving plates.

7. Garnish with chopped tomatoes and fresh parsley.

8. Serve warm.

PER SERVING: CALORIES: 218; CARBS: 12G; GLYCEMIC LOAD: 4; FIBER: 7G; SODIUM: 326MG; PROTEIN: 22G; FAT: 10G; SATURATED FAT: 3G

Coconut Cashew Green Smoothie

DAIRY FREE, GLUTEN FREE
SERVES 2 | PREP TIME: 5 MINUTES

- 1 (13.5-ounce) can light coconut milk
- 1 medium apple, cored and chopped
- 1-inch piece fresh ginger, peeled and minced
- 1 teaspoon ground cinnamon
- 1 teaspoon vanilla extract
- ⅓ cup frozen green peas
- 1 cup stemmed and chopped kale
- 1 cup baby spinach leaves
- ½ cup dry-roasted cashews
- ½ cup ice cubes

1. In a blender, combine the coconut milk, apple, ginger, cinnamon, vanilla, peas, kale, spinach, cashews, and ice.

2. Blend on high until smooth.

3. Immediately pour the mixture into 2 tall glasses and serve.

PER SERVING: CALORIES: 668; CARBS: 38G; GLYCEMIC LOAD: 13; FIBER: 6G; SODIUM: 80MG; PROTEIN: 13G; FAT: 57G; SATURATED FAT: 39G

Almond Flour Muffins

INFLAMMATION FIGHTER, DAIRY FREE, GLUTEN FREE
MAKES 12 | PREP TIME: 5 MINUTES
COOK TIME: 15 TO 20 MINUTES

- **2½ cups almond flour or almond meal**
- **1 teaspoon baking soda**
- **½ teaspoon salt**
- **3 eggs**
- **⅓ cup unsweetened applesauce or pumpkin purée**
- **2 tablespoons agave nectar**
- **2 tablespoons coconut oil, melted**
- **1 teaspoon white vinegar**
- **1 teaspoon vanilla extract**
- **1 cup chopped fresh fruit (optional)**

1. Preheat the oven to 350°F.

2. Line 12 cups of a standard muffin tin with paper liners.

3. In a large bowl, gently whisk together the almond flour, baking soda, and salt.

4. In a medium bowl, whisk together the eggs, applesauce, agave nectar, coconut oil, vinegar, and vanilla.

5. Add the egg mixture to the flour mixture and stir until blended. Fold in the fresh fruit (if using).

6. Divide the batter evenly among the 12 muffin cups in the prepared pan.

7. Bake for 15 to 20 minutes, until the muffins are set at the centers and golden brown on the edges. Transfer to a cooling rack and let cool completely.

8. Store the muffins in a covered container in the refrigerator for up to 1 week or in the freezer for up to 3 months.

PER SERVING: CALORIES: 80; CARBS: 3G; GLYCEMIC LOAD: 2; FIBER: 0G; SODIUM: 217MG; PROTEIN: 3G; FAT: 6G; SATURATED FAT: 2G

Cherry Smoothie Bowl

FERTILITY BOOST, INFLAMMATION FIGHTER, GLUTEN FREE
SERVES 2 | PREP TIME: 5 MINUTES

- 2 cups frozen cherries
- ½ cup old-fashioned rolled oats, soaked in ½ cup unsweetened almond milk overnight
- 1 cup plain nonfat Greek yogurt
- 1 tablespoon chia seeds
- 1 teaspoon vanilla extract
- 1 tablespoon natural almond butter
- 2 teaspoons hemp seeds
- ½ cup fresh berries
- 2 teaspoons sliced almonds

1. In a blender, combine the cherries, soaked oats, yogurt, chia seeds, vanilla, and almond butter. Blend until smooth. Pour into 2 bowls.

2. Top each bowl with 1 teaspoon hemp seeds, ¼ cup fresh berries, and 1 teaspoon sliced almonds. Serve.

PER SERVING: CALORIES: 488; CARBS: 62G; GLYCEMIC LOAD: 26; FIBER: 11G; SODIUM: 128MG; PROTEIN: 18G; FAT: 18G; SATURATED FAT: 3G

Blueberry Muffin Mug Cake

LOWER CALORIE, INFLAMMATION FIGHTER

SERVES 1 | PREP TIME: 5 MINUTES | COOK TIME: 1 TO 2 MINUTES

- 2 tablespoons oat flour
- 1 tablespoon coconut flour
- 1 tablespoon almond flour
- ½ teaspoon baking powder
- ½ teaspoon ground nutmeg
- 1 large egg, lightly beaten
- ½ teaspoon vanilla extract
- 1 tablespoon unsweetened applesauce or pumpkin purée
- 2 tablespoons unsweetened almond milk
- 2 tablespoons frozen blueberries
- Olive oil cooking spray

1. In a large bowl, stir together the oat flour, coconut flour, almond flour, baking powder, and nutmeg.

2. Add the egg, vanilla, applesauce, and almond milk to the flour mixture, and stir until smooth. Gently fold in the blueberries.

3. Coat the sides of a large mug (12 ounces or larger) with olive oil cooking spray. Spoon the batter into the mug.

4. Microwave on high for 50 seconds, then stop and check to see if the batter is set. Continue to microwave, 10 seconds at a time, until the batter is set, about 2 minutes total, depending on the microwave strength.

5. Once the cake is set, let it cool slightly, then transfer it to a plate.

6. Serve warm.

PER SERVING: CALORIES: 308; CARBS: 29G; GLYCEMIC LOAD: 16; FIBER: 1G; SODIUM: 249MG; PROTEIN: 10G; FAT: 18G; SATURATED FAT: 3G

Pumpkin Pie Overnight Oats

LOWER CALORIE, GLUTEN FREE

SERVES 1 | PREP TIME: 5 MINUTES, PLUS 4 HOURS OR MORE TO CHILL

- ½ cup nonfat plain Greek yogurt
- ¼ cup unsweetened pumpkin purée
- 2 tablespoons unsweetened almond milk
- ¼ cup old-fashioned rolled oats
- 1 tablespoon chia seeds
- ½ teaspoon vanilla extract
- ¼ teaspoon ground cinnamon
- ⅛ teaspoon ground nutmeg
- ⅛ teaspoon ground ginger
- Granulated stevia
- 1 tablespoon sliced almonds

1. In a medium bowl or 8-ounce mason jar, combine the yogurt, pumpkin, almond milk, oats, chia seeds, vanilla, cinnamon, nutmeg, ginger, and stevia. Mix thoroughly.

2. Cover and refrigerate for at least 4 hours, or until the oats are soft.

3. Top with the almonds.

PER SERVING: CALORIES: 397; CARBS: 48G; GLYCEMIC LOAD: 21; FIBER: 13G; SODIUM: 95MG; PROTEIN: 18G; FAT: 14G; SATURATED FAT: 3G

Soups and Salads

Mushroom Barley Soup

FERTILITY BOOST, LOWER CALORIE, INFLAMMATION FIGHTER, DAIRY FREE, GLUTEN FREE
SERVES 4 | PREP TIME: 10 MINUTES | COOK TIME: 35 MINUTES

- 1 tablespoon olive oil
- 1 Vidalia onion, thinly sliced
- Salt
- 8 ounces cremini mushrooms, sliced ¼ inch thick
- 2 large portobello mushrooms, cubed
- 1 large carrot, peeled and diced
- 1 medium zucchini, sliced into ¼-inch-thick half moons
- 1 garlic clove, minced
- 3 celery stalks, thinly sliced
- 1 large tomato, diced
- ¾ cups uncooked pearled barley
- 6 cups low-sodium vegetable broth
- Freshly ground black pepper
- 3 tablespoons chopped fresh rosemary leaves, divided
- 3 tablespoons chopped fresh thyme, divided

1. Preheat a 4-quart pot over medium heat. Add the olive oil, onion, and a pinch of salt, and sauté until the onion is softened and translucent, about 5 minutes.

2. Add the mushrooms, carrot, and zucchini, and sauté until the vegetables are slightly softened and some of the moisture has been released, about 5 minutes. Mix in the garlic and sauté for 1 to 2 minutes.

3. Add the celery, tomato, barley, and broth, and season with salt and pepper. Cover and bring the liquid to a boil. Once it's boiling, reduce the heat to low. Stir in 2 tablespoons of the rosemary and 2 tablespoons of the thyme, and return the lid to the pot.

4. Simmer until the barley is tender, about 10 minutes. Taste the soup and season again with salt and pepper as desired. For best results, let the soup sit, covered, for at least 10 minutes so the flavors can blend.

5. Serve the soup garnished with the remaining tablespoons of rosemary and thyme.

PER SERVING: CALORIES: 213; CARBS: 38G; GLYCEMIC LOAD: 16; FIBER: 8G; SODIUM: 902MG; PROTEIN: 8G; FAT: 5G; SATURATED FAT: 1G

Creamy Vegan Kale Soup

INFLAMMATION FIGHTER, DAIRY FREE, GLUTEN FREE

SERVES 4 | PREP TIME: 15 MINUTES, PLUS 4 TO 8 HOURS SOAKING TIME | COOK TIME: 30 MINUTES

- 2 tablespoons olive oil
- 1 medium leek, white and light green parts only, cleaned and sliced
- 4 garlic cloves, minced
- 8 cups low-sodium vegetable broth
- 2 large bunches curly kale, stemmed
- 1 cup raw cashews, soaked in water for 4 to 8 hours, drained and rinsed
- 4 sprigs fresh rosemary
- 4 sprigs fresh thyme
- 2 teaspoons ground nutmeg
- 2 tablespoons white wine vinegar
- ¼ teaspoon salt
- ¼ teaspoon freshly ground black pepper
- ¼ cup roasted pepitas (shelled pumpkin seeds), for garnish

1. Heat the oil in a large Dutch oven over medium heat. Add the leek and garlic and sauté until softened, about 5 minutes. Stir in the broth and remove the pot from the heat.

2. Working in batches, put the kale leaves into a food processor (or blender) and pulse until very finely chopped. Transfer to the pot with the broth.

3. Put the cashews in the food processor (or blender). Blend until smooth, stopping to scrape down the sides of the bowl with a spatula as needed.

4. Transfer the cashew mixture to the pot with the kale and broth, and stir in the rosemary, thyme, and nutmeg. Place the pot over high heat and bring the liquid to a low boil. Reduce the heat to medium low and simmer, uncovered, until the kale is tender, about 10 minutes.

5. Stir in the vinegar, salt, and pepper. Taste and adjust the seasonings as desired.

6. Ladle into bowls and garnish with the pepitas.

PER SERVING: CALORIES: 371; CARBS: 34G; GLYCEMIC LOAD: 11; FIBER: 4G; SODIUM: 829MG; PROTEIN: 12G; FAT: 24G; SATURATED FAT: 4G

Roasted Red Pepper and White Bean Soup

FERTILITY BOOST, INFLAMMATION FIGHTER, DAIRY FREE, GLUTEN FREE
SERVES 4 | PREP TIME: 10 MINUTES | COOK TIME: 30 MINUTES

- 1 tablespoon extra-virgin olive oil, plus more for garnish
- 1 large white onion, diced
- 3 garlic cloves, minced
- 4 medium carrots, peeled and chopped
- 4 cups low-sodium vegetable broth
- 1 (12-ounce) jar roasted red bell peppers, drained and sliced thin, reserving some for garnish
- 1 (15-ounce) can cannellini beans, drained and rinsed
- 1 teaspoon dried basil
- ½ teaspoon dried thyme
- 2 teaspoons paprika
- ½ teaspoon salt
- ¼ cup tahini (sesame paste)

1. Heat the olive oil in a large soup pot over medium heat. Add the onion and garlic and sauté for about 3 minutes, until the onion begins to soften.

2. Add the carrots and sauté for 3 minutes.

3. Add the broth, bell peppers, beans, basil, thyme, paprika, and salt. Increase the heat to high, bring the liquid to a boil, then reduce the heat to low and simmer for 10 to 15 minutes, until the carrots are fork tender.

4. Stir in the tahini, increase the heat to high, bring the soup to a boil, and then immediately remove the pot from the heat.

5. Carefully pour the soup into a blender and purée until smooth.

6. Return the soup to the pot over high heat, and reheat if needed.

7. Ladle the soup into 4 bowls and garnish with a few drizzles of olive oil and a few of the reserved slices of roasted red peppers.

PER SERVING: CALORIES: 312; CARBS: 42G; GLYCEMIC LOAD: 14; FIBER: 9G; SODIUM: 714MG; PROTEIN: 12G; FAT: 12G; SATURATED FAT: 2G

Tuscan Vegetable Soup

FERTILITY BOOST, LOWER CALORIE, DAIRY FREE, GLUTEN FREE
SERVES 4 | PREP TIME: 15 MINUTES | COOK TIME: 25 MINUTES

- 1½ cups peeled and cubed eggplant
- 1 cup water
- 1 (14.5-ounce) can no-salt-added diced tomatoes with their juice
- ½ cup sliced button mushrooms
- 1 portobello mushroom, cubed
- 1 garlic clove, minced
- 1 cup chopped zucchini
- 1 tablespoon chopped fresh thyme (or 1 teaspoon dried)
- 1 tablespoon chopped fresh sage (or ½ teaspoon dried)
- Salt
- Freshly ground black pepper
- 2 packed cups baby spinach leaves

1. In a 3-quart saucepan over high heat, combine the eggplant, water, tomatoes with their juice, button mushrooms, portobello mushroom, garlic, zucchini, thyme, and sage, and season with salt and pepper. Bring to a boil. Cover the pot, reduce the heat to low, and simmer for 20 minutes.

2. Add the spinach and simmer, covered, for an additional 5 minutes or until the vegetables are tender.

3. Ladle into 4 bowls and serve hot.

PER SERVING: CALORIES: 42; CARBS: 8G; GLYCEMIC LOAD: 3; FIBER: 3G; SODIUM: 51MG; PROTEIN: 3G; FAT: 1G; SATURATED FAT: 0G

Black Bean and Chickpea Veggie Chili

INFLAMMATION FIGHTER, DAIRY FREE, GLUTEN FREE
SERVES 4 | PREP TIME: 10 MINUTES | COOK TIME: 35 MINUTES

- 2 tablespoons olive oil
- 1 large white onion, chopped
- Salt
- Freshly ground black pepper
- 2 garlic cloves, minced
- 1 medium green bell pepper, diced
- 2 celery stalks, chopped
- 1 (14.5-ounce) can diced fire-roasted tomatoes and their juice
- 1 (15-ounce) can black beans, drained and rinsed
- 1 (15-ounce) can chickpeas (garbanzo beans), drained and rinsed
- 2 teaspoons ground cumin
- 1½ teaspoons smoked paprika
- 1 teaspoon dried oregano
- 2 tablespoons chili powder
- 2 cups stemmed and chopped kale
- Juice of ½ lime
- 1 green onion (white and light green parts only), chopped, for garnish
- ½ lime, cut into 4 slices, for garnish
- 1 avocado, sliced, for garnish

1. Heat the olive oil in a large soup pot over medium heat. Add the onion, season with salt and pepper, and stir. Sauté until the onion is slightly translucent, about 3 minutes. Then add the garlic, green bell pepper, and celery. Sauté until soft, 5 to 8 minutes. (Turn the heat down to low if the garlic gets too brown.)

2. Add the canned tomatoes and their juice, then fill the can with water and add it to the pot. Stir to combine. Add the beans, chickpeas, cumin, paprika, oregano, chili powder, and kale, and season with salt and pepper. Cover, reduce the heat to low, and cook for 25 minutes, stirring occasionally.

3. Stir in the lime juice.

4. Ladle the chili into 4 bowls and garnish with the green onion, lime slices, and avocado slices.

PER SERVING: CALORIES: 491; CARBS: 71G; GLYCEMIC LOAD: 25; FIBER: 23G; SODIUM: 89MG; PROTEIN: 22G; FAT: 16G; SATURATED FAT: 2G

Spring Vegetable Soup

FERTILITY BOOST, LOWER CALORIE, GLUTEN FREE
SERVES 4 | PREP TIME: 15 MINUTES | COOK TIME: 30 MINUTES

- 2 tablespoons extra-virgin olive oil, divided
- 2 medium carrots, peeled and diced
- 1 large leek, trimmed, cleaned, and chopped
- 1 red bell pepper, diced
- 1 large celery stalk, diced
- 2 garlic cloves, minced
- 5 cups low-sodium vegetable broth
- 1 cup frozen peas
- 10 asparagus spears, cut into 1-inch pieces
- 1 medium zucchini, cut into ¼-inch slices
- 1 (15-ounce) can cannellini beans, drained and rinsed
- 1 teaspoon chopped fresh thyme, plus 1 tablespoon (optional)
- ¼ cup torn fresh basil
- shaved Parmesan cheese (optional for garnish)
- ½ teaspoon salt
- ½ teaspoon freshly ground black pepper

1. Heat a large soup pot or Dutch oven over medium heat. Add 1 tablespoon of the olive oil and swirl to coat. Add the carrots, leek, bell pepper, and celery, stir, and cook, stirring occasionally, for 5 minutes. Add the garlic and cook, stirring, for 1 minute. Increase the heat to high, add the broth, bring the liquid to a boil, then reduce the heat to low and simmer for 5 minutes.

2. Stir in the peas, asparagus, zucchini, and beans. Simmer until the asparagus is crisp tender, 3 to 4 minutes. Add the 1 teaspoon of thyme, and the basil, and stir, cooking for an additional minute.

3. Serve immediately, topped with the remaining tablespoon thyme and Parmesan cheese (if using). Season with the salt and pepper.

PER SERVING: CALORIES: 278; CARBS: 42G; GLYCEMIC LOAD: 14; FIBER: 11G; SODIUM: 765MG; PROTEIN: 12G; FAT: 8G; SATURATED FAT: 1G

Miso Tofu Soup

FERTILITY BOOST, LOWER CALORIE, DAIRY FREE, GLUTEN FREE
SERVES 4 | PREP TIME: 5 MINUTES | COOK TIME: 15 MINUTES

- 5 cups water
- 1 sheet nori (dried seaweed), cut into large rectangles (optional)
- ½ cup chopped green onion (white and light green parts)
- 1 tablespoon peeled and grated fresh ginger
- 1 garlic clove, thinly sliced
- 4 tablespoons white miso paste
- 1 cup chopped green Swiss chard leaves
- 6 ounces firm tofu, drained and cut into ½-inch cubes

1. Bring the water to a boil in a 4-quart pot over medium-high heat. Add the nori (if using), green onion, ginger, and garlic. Reduce the heat to low, cover, and simmer for 10 minutes.

2. In a small bowl, put the miso paste, add a few drops hot water, and whisk until smooth. Stir into the soup.

3. Add the chard and tofu to the pot, return the soup to a gentle simmer, and simmer until the chard is tender, about 5 minutes.

4. Serve immediately.

PER SERVING: CALORIES: 88; CARBS: 9G; GLYCEMIC LOAD: 4; FIBER: 2G; SODIUM: 751MG; PROTEIN: 9G; FAT: 3G; SATURATED FAT: 1G

Broccoli Sprouts Salad with Walnuts and Blueberries

LOWER CALORIE, INFLAMMATION FIGHTER, DAIRY FREE, GLUTEN FREE
SERVES 4 | PREP TIME: 5 MINUTES

2 cups loosely packed fresh broccoli sprouts
1 cup chopped kale leaves
1 cup chopped collard green leaves
½ cup chopped walnuts
½ cup fresh blueberries
Handful fresh cilantro, chopped
1 tablespoon extra-virgin olive oil
Salt
Freshly ground black pepper

1. In a large bowl, combine the sprouts, kale, and collard greens.

2. Add the walnuts, blueberries, cilantro, and olive oil and toss to combine.

3. Season with salt and pepper. Serve immediately.

23G; GLYCEMIC LOAD: 9; FIBER: 2G; SODIUM: 46MG; PROTEIN: 8G; FAT: 14G; SATURATED FAT: 1G

Mason Jar Taco Salad

FERTILITY BOOST, DAIRY FREE, GLUTEN FREE
SERVES 2 | PREP TIME: 10 MINUTES | COOK TIME: 20 MINUTES

- 1 tablespoon extra-virgin olive oil, divided
- 6 ounces boneless skinless chicken breast, cut into bite-size pieces
- 1 large red bell pepper, seeded and sliced
- ½ large white onion, roughly chopped
- 2 teaspoons minced garlic
- 2 teaspoons cumin seeds
- ½ cup canned black beans, drained and rinsed
- Pinch salt
- 1 medium avocado, pitted and cubed
- Juice of 1 large lime
- 4 Roma tomatoes, chopped
- ½ cucumber, peeled and chopped
- ½ cup chopped fresh cilantro
- 2 cups baby spinach leaves

1. In a large skillet, heat ½ tablespoon of the olive oil over medium-high heat. Add the chicken breast and sauté until golden brown, about 8 minutes. Transfer to a small bowl.

2. Add the remaining ½ tablespoon olive oil to the skillet and reduce the heat to medium. Add the bell pepper, onion, and garlic, and sauté until softened and browned, about 5 minutes.

3. In a small, dry pan over medium-high heat, add the cumin seeds, and toast, stirring frequently, until golden brown and fragrant, about 2 minutes. Transfer to a cutting board and crush with the bottom of a sturdy glass.

4. Add the crushed cumin seeds and black beans to the skillet with the veggies, and stir in the salt. Remove the skillet from the heat.

5. Put the avocado and lime juice into a small bowl. Using a fork, mash them together until smooth.

6. To assemble the salads in the mason jars, spread one-fourth of the chopped tomatoes evenly in the bottom of each jar. Put one-fourth of the avocado-lime mixture on top of each, and gently spread out. In each jar, spread a layer of the cumin and roasted veggies, followed by a layer of chicken. Add one-fourth of the remaining tomatoes to each jar, and then add a layer of cucumbers. Finish by adding ¼ cup of the cilantro to each, topped by as much of the spinach as possible.

7. Seal and refrigerate. To eat, turn the jar over and shake to distribute the ingredients. Eat out of the jar, or pour onto a plate.

PER SERVING: CALORIES: 524; CARBS: 44G; GLYCEMIC LOAD: 16; FIBER: 14G; SODIUM: 469MG; PROTEIN: 21G; FAT: 31G; SATURATED FAT: 5G

Chickpea, Tomato, and Basil Salad

LOWER CALORIE, INFLAMMATION FIGHTER, DAIRY FREE, GLUTEN FREE
SERVES 2 TO 4 | PREP TIME: 10 MINUTES, PLUS 20 MINUTES TO CHILL

- **1 (15-ounce) can chickpeas (garbanzo beans), drained and rinsed**
- **1 pint cherry tomatoes, halved**
- **1 cup chopped fresh basil leaves**
- **4 garlic cloves, minced**
- **1 tablespoon red wine vinegar**
- **1 tablespoon apple cider vinegar**
- **2 teaspoons extra-virgin olive oil**
- **½ tablespoon honey**
- **Pinch salt**
- **Freshly ground black pepper**

In a medium bowl, mix together all the ingredients. Chill for about 20 minutes before serving.

PER SERVING: CALORIES: 676; CARBS: 134G; GLYCEMIC LOAD: 67; FIBER: 18G; SODIUM: 75MG; PROTEIN: 21G; FAT: 10G; SATURATED FAT: 1G

Persian Cucumber Salad

LOWER CALORIE, INFLAMMATION FIGHTER, DAIRY FREE, GLUTEN FREE
SERVES 4 | PREP TIME: 10 MINUTES, PLUS 10 MINUTES TO SIT (OR 2 HOURS TO CHILL)

- 5 small Persian cucumbers, unpeeled, or 1 large English cucumber, peeled
- 1½ cups cherry tomatoes
- ½ small red onion
- 3 tablespoons coarsely chopped fresh flat-leaf parsley
- 2 tablespoons coarsely chopped fresh mint
- 1 tablespoon extra-virgin olive oil
- 3 tablespoons freshly squeezed lime juice
- 1 teaspoon freshly grated lime zest
- ⅓ teaspoon coarse sea salt
- ¼ teaspoon freshly ground black pepper

1. Dice the cucumbers, tomatoes, and red onion into small cubes and transfer them to a medium bowl.

2. Add the chopped parsley and mint.

3. In a small bowl, whisk together the olive oil, lime juice, lime zest, salt, pepper, and olive oil.

4. Add the dressing to the salad ingredients and toss gently to coat. Let the salad sit at room temperature for 10 minutes so the flavors can mingle, or cover the bowl and refrigerate for up to 2 hours.

5. Serve chilled.

PER SERVING: CALORIES: 26; CARBS: 6G; GLYCEMIC LOAD: 2; FIBER: 1G; SODIUM: 297MG; PROTEIN: 1G; FAT: 0G; SATURATED FAT: 0G

Artichoke Millet Power Salad

INFLAMMATION FIGHTER, DAIRY FREE, GLUTEN FREE

SERVES 4 | PREP TIME: 10 MINUTES | COOK TIME: 20 MINUTES, PLUS 10 MINUTES (OR UP TO 2 HOURS) TO CHILL

- **2 tablespoons extra-virgin olive oil, divided**
- **2 medium shallots**
- **1 garlic clove, minced**
- **¼ teaspoon salt**
- **½ teaspoon freshly ground black pepper**
- **⅓ cup uncooked millet**
- **⅔ cup water**
- **1 cup finely chopped fresh flat-leaf parsley**
- **¼ cup freshly squeezed lemon juice**
- **2 tablespoons balsamic vinegar**
- **1 pint cherry tomatoes, halved**
- **2 small zucchini, trimmed and chopped**
- **1 (15-ounce) can cannellini beans, drained and rinsed**
- **1 (15-ounce) can artichoke hearts in water, drained and quartered**
- **½ cup roasted pepitas (shelled pumpkin seeds), for garnish**

1. Heat 1 tablespoon of the olive oil in a small saucepan over medium heat. Add the shallots, garlic, salt, and pepper, and sauté until soft and translucent, about 5 minutes.

2. Increase the heat to high and add the millet. While stirring constantly, allow the millet to brown slightly, about 3 minutes.

3. Add the water and bring to a boil. Then reduce the heat to low, cover, and simmer for 10 minutes. Remove the pan from the heat and let the millet steam, covered, for 5 minutes. Transfer to a large bowl and fluff with a fork. Allow to cool slightly.

4. In a medium bowl, combine the chopped parsley, lemon juice, balsamic vinegar, and remaining 1 tablespoon of oil. Massage the mixture together to soften the parsley.

5. To the bowl with the millet mixture, add the tomatoes, zucchini, beans, and artichoke hearts. Add the parsley mixture, and toss until combined.

6. Cover and chill for 10 minutes or up to 2 hours before serving.

7. Serve garnished with the pepitas.

PER SERVING: CALORIES: 433; CARBS: 58G; GLYCEMIC LOAD: 22; FIBER: 19G; SODIUM: 226MG; PROTEIN: 19G; FAT: 16G; SATURATED FAT: 3G

Asian Peanut Slaw

INFLAMMATION FIGHTER, DAIRY FREE, GLUTEN FREE
SERVES 6 | PREP TIME: 10 MINUTES | COOK TIME: 10 MINUTES

- **1 (12-ounce) bag non-GMO frozen shelled edamame**
- 3 cups shredded green cabbage
- 2 cups shredded carrots
- 1 cup shredded purple cabbage
- 1 cup chopped fresh cilantro
- 1 cup green onions, chopped (white and light green parts)
- 1 cup roasted unsalted peanuts
- ⅓ cup extra-virgin olive oil
- 3 tablespoons rice vinegar
- 1 tablespoon sesame oil
- 1 teaspoon Bragg's liquid aminos
- 1 teaspoon ground ginger
- 1 teaspoon honey

1. Place the edamame in a medium saucepan over medium-high heat, cover with water, and cook until tender, about 8 minutes. Drain in a colander.

2. Meanwhile, in a large bowl, combine the green cabbage, carrots, purple cabbage, cilantro, green onions, and peanuts.

3. In a small bowl, whisk together the olive oil, rice vinegar, sesame oil, aminos, ginger, and honey until the mixture is emulsified.

4. Add the dressing and cooked edamame to the cabbage mixture and toss until thoroughly combined.

5. Serve immediately.

PER SERVING: CALORIES: 378; CARBS: 21G; GLYCEMIC LOAD: 5; FIBER: 8G; SODIUM: 103MG; PROTEIN: 11G; FAT: 30G; SATURATED FAT: 4G

Almond Chicken and Greens Soup

INFLAMMATION FIGHTER, DAIRY FREE, GLUTEN FREE
SERVES 4 | PREP TIME: 10 MINUTES | COOK TIME: 30 MINUTES

- 4 cups low-sodium chicken broth
- ½ small yellow onion, diced
- 2 garlic cloves, minced
- 1 red bell pepper, diced
- 1 large sweet potato, peeled and diced
- 8 ounces boneless, skinless chicken breast, cut into bite-size pieces
- ½ cup natural creamy almond butter
- 2 cups stemmed and thinly sliced kale
- 2 tablespoons peeled and minced fresh ginger
- Salt
- Freshly ground black pepper
- 1 lime, cut into 4 wedges

1. In a 4-quart pot over medium-high heat, combine the broth, onion, garlic, bell pepper, and sweet potato and bring to a boil. Reduce the heat to low. Add the chicken, cover, and simmer for 20 minutes or until the chicken is cooked through.

2. In a small bowl, whisk together the almond butter and ½ cup of the soup mixture into a thick paste. Set aside.

3. Add the kale and ginger to the soup, and stir to combine. Increase the heat to high and bring the liquid to a boil; then reduce the heat to low and simmer, covered, for 5 minutes. Stir in the almond butter paste and season with salt and pepper.

4. Ladle the soup into 4 soup bowls and squeeze each with a lime wedge.

PER SERVING: CALORIES: 421; CARBS: 32G; GLYCEMIC LOAD: 9; FIBER: 4G; SODIUM: 841MG; PROTEIN: 15G; FAT: 28G; SATURATED FAT: 4G

Vegetable Quinoa Mega Bowl

INFLAMMATION FIGHTER, DAIRY FREE, GLUTEN FREE
SERVES 6 | PREP TIME: 25 MINUTES | COOK TIME: 20 MINUTES

FOR THE DRESSING

⅓ cup natural almond butter

⅓ cup extra-virgin olive oil

3 garlic cloves, minced (approximately 1 tablespoon)

3-inch piece fresh ginger, peeled and minced (1 to 2 tablespoons)

Juice of 3 limes (approximately ⅓ cup)

Water, to thin

FOR THE VEGETABLE QUINOA

1 cup uncooked quinoa

2 cups water

½ head red cabbage, shredded (approximately 3 cups)

½ cup diced green onions

½ cup fresh cilantro, chopped

1 (15-ounce) can navy beans, drained and rinsed

1 cup diced zucchini

¾ cup chopped almonds

TO MAKE THE DRESSING

Put all of the ingredients in a food processor (or blender) and blend until smooth. Add water, a few drops at a time, as needed to thin until desired consistency.

TO MAKE THE VEGETABLE QUINOA

1. In a medium saucepan over medium-high heat, combine the quinoa and the water. Bring to a rolling boil and let it cook for 1 minute; then reduce the heat to low, cover the pan, and cook for 15 minutes, until the quinoa absorbs the water.

2. Remove the pan from the heat and let it stand for 5 minutes, covered. Remove the lid and fluff gently with a fork. Transfer to a large mixing bowl.

3. Add the cabbage, green onions, cilantro, beans, zucchini, and almonds, and stir to combine. Pour the dressing over the quinoa-veggie mixture and toss until the ingredients are all well coated.

4. Distribute into 6 bowls and serve immediately. Or place in an airtight container and refrigerate for up to 3 days.

PER SERVING: CALORIES: 533; CARBS: 50G; GLYCEMIC LOAD: 18; FIBER: 15G; SODIUM: 21MG; PROTEIN: 19G; FAT: 31G; SATURATED FAT: 3G

Moroccan Spiced Buckwheat Salad

INFLAMMATION FIGHTER, DAIRY TREE, GLUTEN FREE
SERVES 4 | PREP TIME: 10 MINUTES

- 2 cups cooked buckwheat
- 1 (15-ounce) can chickpeas (garbanzo beans), drained and rinsed
- 1 small red onion, chopped
- 2 cups stemmed, thinly sliced kale
- 1 cup chopped carrots
- 4 dried apricots, finely chopped
- 2 green onions, sliced (white and light green parts)
- ¼ cup chopped fresh cilantro
- 2 tablespoons extra-virgin olive oil
- ⅓ cup rice wine vinegar
- 3 teaspoons ground cumin
- ½ teaspoon salt
- ¼ cup sunflower seeds (optional)

1. In a large bowl, stir together the buckwheat, chick-peas, red onion, kale, carrots, apricots, green onions, and cilantro.

2. In a small bowl, whisk the olive oil, vinegar, cumin, and salt until combined.

3. Add the dressing to the buckwheat and vegetable mixture, and toss until coated.

4. Serve topped with the sunflower seeds (if using).

PER SERVING: CALORIES: 359; CARBS: 56G; GLYCEMIC LOAD: 22; FIBER: 13G; SODIUM: 342MG; PROTEIN: 14G; FAT: 10G; SATURATED FAT: 1G

Snacks and Sides

Lentil-Stuffed Avocado

INFLAMMATION FIGHTER, DAIRY FREE, GLUTEN FREE
SERVES 4 | PREP TIME: 5 MINUTES | COOK TIME: 35 MINUTES

½ cup dry lentils
1 tablespoon extra-virgin olive oil
1 small white onion, halved and sliced
2 garlic cloves, chopped
10 cherry tomatoes, halved
⅛ teaspoon smoked paprika
Salt
Freshly ground black pepper
2 large avocados
2 tablespoons chopped fresh cilantro (optional)

1. Bring 2 cups of water to a boil in a medium saucepan over high heat. Stir in the lentils, and cook for 15 minutes. Drain.

2. Meanwhile, in a medium saucepan over medium heat, add the onion and sauté until translucent, about 3 minutes. Add the garlic and sauté for 1 minute.

3. Add the tomatoes and smoked paprika, season with salt and pepper, and stir to combine. Simmer for 10 minutes, stirring frequently. Taste and adjust the seasoning for salt and pepper.

4. Add the lentils to the vegetable mixture, stir, and cook for 2 to 3 minutes.

5. Cut the avocados in half, and core. Put the halves on 4 plates. Top with the lentil mixture and top with the chopped cilantro (if using).

PER SERVING: CALORIES: 312; CARBS: 30G; GLYCEMIC LOAD: 12; FIBER: 12G; SODIUM: 33MG; PROTEIN: 10G; FAT: 19G; SATURATED FAT: 4G

Mushroom Hummus Dippers

FERTILITY BOOST, DAIRY FREE, GLUTEN FREE
SERVES 6 | PREP TIME: 10 MINUTES | COOK TIME: 15 MINUTES

3 cups baby bello or portobello mushrooms, sliced
⅓ cup olive oil, plus 2 tablespoons
Salt
Freshly ground black pepper
1 (15-ounce) can chickpeas (garbanzo beans), drained and rinsed
⅓ cup tahini (sesame paste)
2 garlic cloves, minced
Juice of 1 lemon
Water
1 tablespoon chopped fresh flat-leaf parsley

1. Preheat the oven to 425°F.

2. Line a baking sheet with aluminum foil.

3. Layer the sliced mushrooms on the prepared pan, drizzle with ⅓ cup of the olive oil, and season with salt and pepper. Roast for 15 minutes until browned, stirring them halfway through. Set aside on a cooling rack.

4. In a food processor (or blender), add the remaining 2 tablespoons olive oil, chickpeas, tahini, garlic, and lemon juice. Pulse for a few seconds, adding a few drops of water as needed to thin the mixture. Add the mushrooms and pulse again, adding a few drops of water until the desired consistency is reached. Season with salt and pepper.

5. Portion into 6 mason jars or another airtight container. Refrigerate for up to 4 days.

PER SERVING: CALORIES: 332; CARBS: 26G; GLYCEMIC LOAD: 9; FIBER: 8G; SODIUM: 45MG; PROTEIN: 11G; FAT: 23G; SATURATED FAT: 2G

Real Food Vegan Protein Bars

GLUTEN FREE, DAIRY FREE
SERVES 10 | PREP TIME: 10 MINUTES | COOK TIME: 30 MINUTES

- **Olive oil cooking spray**
- **½ cup old-fashioned rolled oats**
- **2 tablespoons chia seeds**
- **⅓ cup (about 8) dried apricots, roughly chopped**
- **1¾ cups canned chickpeas (garbanzo beans), drained and rinsed**
- **3 tablespoons honey**
- **2 tablespoons hemp seeds**
- **⅔ cup unsweetened almond or coconut milk**
- **1 teaspoon vanilla extract**
- **1 teaspoon ground cinnamon**

1. Preheat the oven to 350°F.

2. Coat a 9-by-9-inch baking pan with olive oil cooking spray.

3. In a blender, combine the oats, chia seeds, and apricots, and blend until chopped. Pour into a large mixing bowl.

4. In the blender, add the chickpeas and blend until chopped but not puréed, with a texture similar to oatmeal. Add to the oats mixture.

5. To the oats mixture, add the honey, hemp seeds, almond milk, vanilla, and cinnamon and mix well.

6. Add the batter to the prepared pan and press down so it is even on top.

7. Bake for about 30 minutes, or until the edges are golden brown and the center is no longer soft.

8. Cool in the pan on a cooling rack. Cut into squares. Store in an airtight container in the refrigerator for up to 4 days, or in a resealable plastic bag in the freezer for up to 3 months.

PER SERVING: CALORIES: 164; CARBS: 22G; GLYCEMIC LOAD: 10; FIBER: 4G; SODIUM: 5MG; PROTEIN: 6G; FAT: 7G; SATURATED FAT: 3G

Portable Paella Cups

INFLAMMATION FIGHTER, DAIRY FREE, GLUTEN FREE
SERVES 8 | PREP TIME: 20 MINUTES | COOK TIME: 30 MINUTES

- 1 cup water
- ¼ cup chickpea flour (you can substitute almond flour)
- 1 tablespoon olive oil
- 1 tablespoon flaxseed meal
- 2 garlic cloves, minced
- ¾ teaspoon ground turmeric
- ¾ teaspoon salt
- 2 cups cooked and cooled brown rice
- ⅔ cup canned chickpeas (garbanzo beans), drained and rinsed
- ½ cup frozen green peas, thawed
- ½ cup roasted red peppers, chopped
- ⅓ cup artichoke hearts, drained and chopped

1. Preheat the oven to 350°F.

2. Line 8 cups of a standard muffin tin with paper liners.

3. In a large bowl, whisk together the water, chickpea flour, olive oil, flaxseed meal, garlic, turmeric, salt, and pepper until blended. Stir in the rice, chickpeas, peas, red peppers, and artichoke hearts. Mix thoroughly to combine.

4. Divide the mixture evenly among the prepared muffin cups.

5. Bake for 25 to 30 minutes until the centers feel set and tops appear golden and crispy.

6. Cool completely in the tin. Remove the paella cups.

7. Serve at room temperature, cold, or rewarmed in the microwave for 15 to 30 seconds.

PER SERVING: CALORIES: 128; CARBS: 21G; GLYCEMIC LOAD: 9; FIBER: 4G; SODIUM: 241MG; PROTEIN: 4G; FAT: 3G; SATURATED FAT: 0G

"Cheesy" Baked Spinach Chips

LOWER CALORIE, INFLAMMATION FIGHTER, DAIRY FREE
SERVES 4 | PREP TIME: 5 MINUTES | COOK TIME: 25 MINUTES

- **2 cups baby spinach**
- **1 tablespoon olive oil**
- **3 tablespoons nutritional yeast, divided**
- **¼ teaspoon garlic powder**
- **Salt**
- **Freshly ground black pepper**

1. Preheat the oven to 325°F.

2. Line 2 baking sheets with parchment paper.

3. In a medium bowl, combine the spinach, olive oil, and 2 tablespoons of the nutritional yeast, and gently toss until all of the spinach leaves are coated.

4. Lay the spinach leaves in a single layer on the prepared baking sheets. Sprinkle with the garlic powder, salt, pepper, and the remaining 1 tablespoon nutritional yeast.

5. Bake for 12 minutes; then turn the oven off and leave the pans in the oven for an additional 5 minutes.

6. Remove the pans from the oven and let the spinach sit for 5 minutes more to crisp up.

7. Once completely cooled, store in an airtight bag for 2 to 3 days. The crispy texture will begin to fade after 24 hours, so enjoy these right after baking as possible.

PER SERVING: CALORIES: 51; CARBS: 3G; GLYCEMIC LOAD: 1; FIBER: 2G; SODIUM: 38MG; PROTEIN: 3G; FAT: 4G; SATURATED FAT: 0G

Garlicky Roasted Edamame

LOWER CALORIE, INFLAMMATION FIGHTER, DAIRY FREE, GLUTEN FREE

MAKES ABOUT 22 (¼ CUP) SERVINGS | PREP TIME: 5 MINUTES COOK TIME: 50 MINUTES

Olive oil cooking spray
1 pound non-GMO frozen, shelled edamame, thawed
½ teaspoon salt
½ teaspoon freshly ground black pepper
½ teaspoon garlic powder
1½ teaspoons olive oil

1. Preheat the oven to 400°F.

2. Lightly coat a baking sheet with olive oil cooking spray.

3. In a medium bowl, toss the edamame with the salt, pepper, garlic, and olive oil.

4. Spread out on the prepared pan, and roast for 50 to 60 minutes or until golden brown.

5. Cool completely. Store in an airtight container at room temperature for up to 4 days.

PER SERVING: CALORIES: 25; CARBS: 2G; GLYCEMIC LOAD: 1; FIBER: 1G; SODIUM: 54MG; PROTEIN: 2G; FAT: 1G; SATURATED FAT: 0G

No-Bake Mini Stuffed Peppers

LOWER CALORIE, INFLAMMATION FIGHTER, GLUTEN FREE
MAKES 30 | PREP TIME: 20 MINUTES

- **1 (24 to 32-ounce) bag mini bell peppers**
- **1 (15-ounce) can chickpeas (garbanzo beans), drained and rinsed**
- **¼ cup plain, unsweetened Greek yogurt**
- **1 tablespoon apple cider vinegar**
- **½ teaspoon mustard powder**
- **½ teaspoon dried thyme**
- **2 green onions, sliced thinly**
- **½ teaspoon salt**
- **Pinch cayenne pepper**

1. Cut the stems off of the peppers. Slice lengthwise. Remove any seeds that are inside. Set aside.

2. In the bowl of a food processor (or blender), put the chickpeas, yogurt, vinegar, mustard, thyme, and green onions, salt, and cayenne pepper.

3. Pulse 4 or 5 times. The chickpeas should still be a bit chunky.

4. Remove the blade and stir to make sure the mixture is blended well.

5. Stuff each pepper half with about 2 tablespoons of the chickpea mixture.

6. Serve, or store in an airtight container in the refrigerator for up to 3 days.

PER SERVING: CALORIES: 34; CARBS: 6G; GLYCEMIC LOAD: 2; FIBER: 2G; SODIUM: 43MG; PROTEIN: 2G; FAT: 0G; SATURATED FAT: 0G

"Cheesy" Popcorn

LOWER CALORIE, INFLAMMATION FIGHTER, DAIRY FREE, GLUTEN FREE
SERVES 3 | PREP TIME: 5 MINUTES | COOK TIME: 10 MINUTES

- 2 tablespoons nutritional yeast
- ⅛ teaspoon ground turmeric
- ¼ to ½ teaspoon sea salt
- ¼ teaspoon paprika (optional)
- ¼ teaspoon garlic powder (optional)
- ¼ teaspoon onion powder (optional)
- ⅛ teaspoon cayenne pepper (optional)
- 1 tablespoon coconut oil (preferred because of its high smoke point)
- ¼ cup organic corn kernels

1. In a small bowl, add the nutritional yeast, turmeric, salt, and your choice of optional spices. Stir to combine and set aside.

2. In a large lidded saucepan over high heat, add the coconut oil and heat till it melts and is hot.

3. Add 2 to 3 corn kernels and cover the pan with a lid. Shake the pot a little and wait for all 3 to pop. When they do, remove the lid carefully (be careful of the steam), and remove the kernels with a spoon.

4. Add the remaining corn kernels and cover the pan with a lid.

5. Keep the heat on high and shake the pot, holding the lid down so there's no steam escaping.

6. When the corn starts popping, shake the pot every 3 to 5 seconds so the popcorn doesn't burn.

7. When there are 5-second gaps between popping, remove the pan from the heat immediately. Don't try to pop every kernel or you will burn the popcorn.

8. Carefully remove the lid and transfer the popcorn to a big bowl. Sprinkle with the seasoning mix, and toss to coat quickly and well.

9. Serve immediately.

PER SERVING: CALORIES: 124; CARBS: 16G; GLYCEMIC LOAD: 8; FIBER: 4G; SODIUM: 391MG; PROTEIN: 5G; FAT: 5G; SATURATED FAT: 4G

Roasted Vegetables

LOWER CALORIE, INFLAMMATION FIGHTER, DAIRY FREE, GLUTEN FREE
SERVES 6 | PREP TIME: 15 MINUTES | COOK TIME: 15 MINUTES

- **2 tablespoons extra-virgin olive oil, plus more for the pan**
- **2 cups bite-size broccoli florets**
- **2 cups button mushrooms**
- **1 cup diced butternut squash**
- **2 cups chopped green beans (2-inch pieces)**
- **1 zucchini, quartered lengthwise and cut into 2-inch pieces**
- **1 yellow summer squash, diced**
- **1 red bell pepper, diced**
- **1 red onion, chopped**
- **2 tablespoons balsamic vinegar**
- **4 garlic cloves, minced**
- **2 teaspoons dried rosemary**
- **1½ teaspoons dried thyme**
- **Salt**
- **Freshly ground black pepper**

1. Preheat the oven to 425°F.

2. Lightly coat a baking sheet with olive oil.

3. In the prepared pan, spread the broccoli, mushrooms, squash, green beans, zucchini, squash, bell pepper, and red onion in a single layer.

4. Sprinkle the vegetables with the 2 tablespoons olive oil, the balsamic vinegar, garlic, rosemary, and thyme, and season with salt and pepper. Gently toss to combine.

5. Bake for 12 to 15 minutes, or until all the veggies are fork tender.

6. Serve immediately.

PER SERVING: CALORIES: 92; CARBS: 11G; GLYCEMIC LOAD: 4; FIBER: 3G; SODIUM: 33MG; PROTEIN: 3G; FAT: 5G; SATURATED FAT: 1G

Garlic-Lemon Swiss Chard and Butter Beans

FERTILITY BOOST, LOWER CALORIE, INFLAMMATION FIGHTER, DAIRY FREE, GLUTEN FREE
SERVES 2 TO 3 | PREP TIME: 5 MINUTES | COOK TIME: 10 MINUTES

- **1 large bunch Swiss chard, washed and shaken dry**
- **2 teaspoons extra-virgin olive oil, plus more if needed**
- **2 teaspoons minced garlic**
- **1 (15-ounce) can butter beans, drained and rinsed (or an equal amount cooked fresh or frozen lima beans)**
- **2 tablespoons freshly squeezed lemon juice, plus more if needed**
- **Salt**
- **Freshly ground black pepper**

1. Slice each chard leaf lengthwise on both sides of the stem. Discard the stems (or save them for another use). Stack the chard leaves and cut them crosswise into ¾-inch-thick strips.

2. Heat the olive oil in a large pot over medium heat, swirling the pan to coat. When the oil begins to shimmer, add the garlic and stir for about 30 seconds until fragrant and light brown.

3. Stir in the chard, cover the pot, reduce the heat to medium low, and cook for 5 minutes or until the chard has wilted.

4. Remove the lid from the pot and gently stir in the beans and lemon juice; season with salt and pepper. Cook for 4 to 5 minutes, stirring occasionally. Add a drizzle of olive oil if the beans start to dry out.

5. Taste and add more lemon juice, salt, and/or pepper if desired. Serve hot.

PER SERVING: CALORIES: 295; CARBS: 46G; GLYCEMIC LOAD: 19; FIBER: 13G; SODIUM: 290MG; PROTEIN: 18G; FAT: 6G; SATURATED FAT: 1G

Portobello Eggs with Sun-Dried Tomatoes

FERTILITY BOOST, LOWER CALORIE, DAIRY FREE, GLUTEN FREE
SERVES 2 | PREP TIME: 5 MINUTES | COOK TIME: 15 MINUTES

- **2 portobello mushroom caps**
- **Olive oil cooking spray**
- **2 tablespoons finely chopped sun-dried tomatoes (not packed in oil)**
- **2 eggs**
- **⅛ teaspoon garlic powder**
- **Salt**
- **Freshly ground black pepper**
- **¼ cup chopped fresh basil, for garnish**

1. Preheat the oven to 400°F. Line a baking sheet with aluminum foil.

2. Remove the stems from the mushroom caps and scrape out the gills with a spoon.

3. Coat both sides of the mushroom caps with olive oil cooking spray, or lightly brush them with olive oil, and set them upside-down on the prepared baking sheet.

4. Sprinkle the sun-dried tomatoes into the mushroom caps, dividing them equally.

5. Crack an egg into each mushroom cap, attempting to get the yolk to sit in the cavity where you removed the stem so it stays in place.

6. Carefully transfer the baking sheet to the oven, and bake for 15 minutes or until the egg whites are opaque and the eggs have set.

7. Remove the baking sheet from the oven and season the mushrooms with the garlic powder, salt, and pepper.

8. Sprinkle with the basil and serve hot.

PER SERVING: CALORIES: 124; CARBS: 8G; GLYCEMIC LOAD: 4; FIBER: 3G; SODIUM: 208MG; PROTEIN: 12G; FAT: 6G; SATURATED FAT: 2G

Shredded Brussels Sprouts with Nuts and Berries

FERTILITY BOOST, LOWER CALORIE, INFLAMMATION FIGHTER, DAIRY FREE, GLUTEN FREE
SERVES 8 | PREP TIME: 15 MINUTES | COOK TIME: 10 MINUTES

- **1 pound Brussels sprouts, trimmed**
- **2 teaspoons extra-virgin olive oil, divided**
- **½ red onion, diced**
- **⅓ cup shelled pistachios, roughly chopped**
- **½ cup fresh cranberries**
- **1 tablespoon hemp seeds**
- **Salt**
- **½ teaspoon freshly ground black pepper**

1. Cut each Brussels sprout in half through the stem, and cut into thin slices.

2. Heat 1 teaspoon of the olive oil in a large skillet over medium heat. Add the onion and cook, stirring occasionally, until it begins to soften, 4 to 5 minutes.

3. Add the remaining 1 teaspoon olive oil to the skillet, and then add the Brussels sprouts. Cook, stirring occasionally, until the Brussels sprouts are almost tender but still bright green.

4. Stir in the pistachios, cranberries, and hemp seeds, and season with salt and add the pepper.

5. Serve immediately.

PER SERVING: CALORIES: 113; CARBS: 12G; GLYCEMIC LOAD: 5; FIBER: 3G; SODIUM: 27MG; PROTEIN: 4G; FAT: 7G; SATURATED FAT: 1G

Crispy Baked Zucchini Fries

FERTILITY BOOST, LOWER CALORIE, DAIRY FREE, GLUTEN FREE
SERVES 2 | PREP TIME: 15 MINUTES | COOK TIME: 20 MINUTES

- **Olive oil cooking spray**
- **2 medium zucchini, trimmed**
- **2 egg whites**
- **½ cup whole-wheat panko bread crumbs (see Ingredient Tip)**
- **½ teaspoon dried rosemary**
- **¾ teaspoon garlic powder**
- **¾ teaspoon onion powder**
- **⅛ teaspoon salt**
- **⅛ teaspoon freshly ground black pepper**

1. Preheat the oven to 350°F.

2. Spray a large baking sheet with olive oil cooking spray.

3. Cut the zucchini into long spears.

4. Put the zucchini spears in a large bowl. Add the egg whites, and toss gently to coat.

5. In a medium-large bowl, combine the bread crumbs, rosemary, garlic powder, onion powder, salt, and pepper.

6. One at a time, shake zucchini spears to remove excess egg, and lightly coat with bread crumb mixture. Place each spear on the baking sheet, leaving a bit of space between them. Sprinkle with the remaining bread crumbs.

7. Bake for 10 minutes. Carefully flip the spears and bake for an additional 10 minutes until lightly browned and crispy.

8. Let cool for 10 minutes. Serve hot.

PER SERVING: CALORIES: 177; CARBS: 30G; GLYCEMIC LOAD: 19; FIBER: 2G; SODIUM: 376MG; PROTEIN: 9G; FAT: 2G; SATURATED FAT: 0G

Sesame Asparagus

FERTILITY BOOST, LOWER CALORIE, DAIRY FREE, GLUTEN FREE
SERVES 4 | PREP TIME: 5 MINUTES | COOK TIME: 10 MINUTES

- **1 bunch fresh asparagus, trimmed**
- **1 tablespoon extra-virgin olive oil**
- **Salt**
- **2 tablespoons black sesame seeds, lightly toasted (see Cooking Tip)**
- **Freshly ground black pepper**

1. Fill a large saucepan with ½ inch of water and bring it to a boil over medium heat. Add the asparagus and cook until tender crisp, about 5 minutes, being careful not to overcook. Carefully drain the asparagus and rinse it under cold water. Drain well and transfer to a plate.

2. Return the pan to the stove over medium heat, add the olive oil, and swirl it in the bottom of the pan to coat.

3. Add the asparagus to the pan, shaking off any excess water. Season with salt and pepper and toss with the toasted sesame seeds. Cook the asparagus over medium heat until it is warmed through.

4. Serve immediately.

PER SERVING: CALORIES: 81; CARBS: 4G; GLYCEMIC LOAD: 1; FIBER: 2G; SODIUM: 26MG; PROTEIN: 3G; FAT: 7G; SATURATED FAT: 1G

Roasted Brussels Sprouts, Red Onion, and Apple

FERTILITY BOOST, LOWER CALORIE, INFLAMMATION FIGHTER, DAIRY FREE, GLUTEN FREE
SERVES 4 | PREP TIME: 10 MINUTES | COOK TIME: 15 MINUTES

- **Olive oil cooking spray**
- **1 pound Brussels sprouts, fairly equal in size, trimmed**
- **2 medium red onions, cut into 2-inch chunks**
- **2 medium Yellow Delicious apples, cored and cut into 2-inch chunks**
- **2 tablespoons extra-virgin olive oil**
- **1 tablespoon minced garlic**
- **1 teaspoon mustard powder**
- **1 teaspoon smoked paprika**
- **1 teaspoon salt**
- **¼ teaspoon freshly ground black pepper**

1. Preheat the oven to 400°F.

2. Lightly coat a baking sheet with olive oil cooking spray.

3. Put the Brussels sprouts in a large, microwave-safe mixing bowl and heat them on high for 3 minutes.

4. Remove the Brussels sprouts from the microwave and add the onions, apples, olive oil, garlic, mustard, paprika, and salt, and toss to combine.

5. On each skewer, alternate the Brussels sprouts with red onion and apple in any order you prefer, leaving about ½ inch between each food item.

6. Place the skewers on the prepared baking sheet. Roast for 10 to 15 minutes until the Brussels sprouts, onions, and apples are crisp on the outside and tender on the inside.

7. Add the black pepper and serve hot.

PER SERVING: CALORIES: 178; CARBS: 28G; GLYCEMIC LOAD: 8; FIBER: 7G; SODIUM: 613MG; PROTEIN: 5G; FAT: 7G; SATURATED FAT: 1G

Vegetarian and Vegan Entrées

Cauliflower Fried Rice

LOWER CALORIE, INFLAMMATION FIGHTER, DAIRY FREE, GLUTEN FREE
SERVES 4 | PREP TIME: 10 MINUTES | COOK TIME: 10 MINUTES

- 24 ounces (about 5 cups) cauliflower florets
- 2 tablespoons Bragg's liquid aminos
- 1 tablespoon toasted sesame oil
- 1 tablespoon peeled and minced fresh ginger
- ¼ teaspoon freshly ground white pepper
- 2 teaspoons plus 1 tablespoon olive oil, divided
- 2 eggs, beaten
- 2 garlic cloves, minced
- 1 medium white onion, diced
- ½ cup bite-size broccoli florets
- 1 red bell pepper, chopped
- 2 medium carrots, peeled and grated
- 1 cup snow peas
- 2 green onions, thinly sliced (white and light green parts)
- 1 teaspoon sesame seeds

1. To make the cauliflower rice, put the cauliflower in the bowl of a food processor (or blender) and pulse until it resembles rice, 2 to 3 minutes; set aside.

2. In a small bowl, whisk together the aminos, sesame oil, ginger, and white pepper; set aside.

3. Heat 2 teaspoons of the olive oil in a medium skillet over low heat. Swirl the oil in the pan so it coats the bottom. Add the eggs and cook, 2 to 3 minutes per side, flipping only once. Let cool, then chop into small pieces and set aside on a plate.

4. Heat the remaining tablespoon of olive oil in a large skillet or wok over medium-high heat. Add the garlic and onion and cook, stirring often, until the onion has become translucent, 3 to 4 minutes. Stir in the broccoli, bell pepper, carrots, and snow peas. Cook, stirring constantly, until the vegetables are crisp tender, 3 to 4 minutes.

5. Stir in the cauliflower, chopped eggs, green onions, and aminos mixture. Cook, stirring constantly, until everything is heated through and the cauliflower is tender, 3 to 4 minutes.

6. Serve hot, garnished with the sesame seeds.

PER SERVING: CALORIES: 195; CARBS: 21G; GLYCEMIC LOAD: 9; FIBER: 8G; SODIUM: 618MG; PROTEIN: 10G; FAT: 9G; SATURATED FAT: 2G

Mini Crustless Quiches

FERTILITY BOOSTING, LOWER CALORIE, DAIRY FREE, GLUTEN FREE
MAKES 12 SMALL OR 6 LARGER QUICHES
PREP TIME: 10 MINUTES | COOK TIME: 15 MINUTES

Olive oil cooking spray
1 tablespoon olive oil
½ cup finely chopped white onion
½ cup finely chopped mushrooms
½ cup finely chopped green bell pepper
¼ cup finely chopped tomatoes
1 cup frozen and thawed spinach or kale
6 eggs
½ teaspoon dried thyme
¼ cup nutritional yeast (optional)
Salt
Freshly ground black pepper

1. Preheat the oven to 350°F.

2. Coat the cups of a standard 12-cup muffin tin with olive oil cooking spray.

3. Heat the olive oil in a large skillet over medium heat. Add the onion, mushrooms, bell pepper, tomatoes, and spinach and sauté until the vegetables have softened, about 5 minutes. Remove the skillet from the heat.

4. Whisk the eggs in a medium bowl. Add the thyme and nutritional yeast (if using), and season with salt and pepper. Stir in the sautéed veggies.

5. Fill each of the prepared muffin cups ¾ of the way to the top with the egg mixture (this recipe makes 12 low or 6 taller quiches).

6. Bake for 10 to 15 minutes for low quiches or 15 to 20 minutes for taller quiches. They are done when the egg mixture has set and is firm to the touch.

7. Remove the quiches from the oven and let them cool slightly.

8. Serve warm or wrap the quiches in plastic and refrigerate for up to 3 days.

PER SERVING: CALORIES: 51; CARBS: 1G; GLYCEMIC LOAD: 1; FIBER: 0G; SODIUM: 38MG; PROTEIN: 3G; FAT: 4G; SATURATED FAT: 1G

One-Pan Asparagus Eggs

FERTILITY BOOST, LOWER CALORIE, INFLAMMATION FIGHTER, DAIRY FREE, GLUTEN FREE
SERVES 4 | PREP TIME: 5 MINUTES | COOK TIME: 20 MINUTES

- **Olive oil cooking spray**
- **1 pound asparagus, trimmed**
- **1 pint cherry tomatoes**
- **1 tablespoon extra-virgin olive oil**
- **2 garlic cloves, minced**
- **¼ cup chopped fresh basil leaves**
- **Salt**
- **Freshly ground black pepper**
- **4 eggs**

1. Preheat the oven to 400°F. Coat a baking sheet with olive oil cooking spray.

2. Arrange the asparagus and cherry tomatoes in an even layer on the prepared baking sheet. Drizzle the olive oil over the vegetables. Sprinkle with the garlic and basil, and season with salt and pepper.

3. Roast until the asparagus is nearly tender and the tomatoes are wrinkled, 10 to 12 minutes.

4. Crack the eggs on top of the vegetables, and season each with salt and pepper.

5. Bake until the egg whites are set and the yolks are still soft, 7 to 8 minutes.

6. Remove the baking sheet from the oven and divide the asparagus, tomatoes, and eggs among 4 plates; serve hot.

PER SERVING: CALORIES: 133; CARBS: 7G; GLYCEMIC LOAD: 3; FIBER: 3G; SODIUM: 99MG; PROTEIN: 9G; FAT: 9G; SATURATED FAT: 2G

Almond-Crusted Tofu

INFLAMMATION FIGHTER, DAIRY FREE, GLUTEN FREE
SERVES 4 | PREP TIME: 30 MINUTES | COOK TIME: 25 MINUTES

- **2 egg whites**
- **1 cup almond meal**
- **½ teaspoon paprika**
- **½ teaspoon garlic powder**
- **½ teaspoon salt**
- **½ teaspoon freshly ground black pepper**
- **1 (15- or 16-ounce) block organic extra-firm tofu, cut into 12 squares, drained and patted dry**

1. Preheat the oven to 375°F. Line a baking sheet with parchment paper.

2. In a small shallow bowl, whisk the egg whites.

3. In another small shallow bowl, whisk together the almond meal, paprika, garlic powder, salt, and pepper.

4. Dip each square of tofu into the egg whites, letting the excess fall back into the dish.

5. Press all sides of each tofu square into the almond meal mixture to coat. Place the coated tofu squares on the prepared baking sheet, cover, and refrigerate for at least 20 minutes to set the crust.

6. Bake for approximately 20 to 25 minutes until golden and crispy.

7. Serve immediately.

PER SERVING: CALORIES: 104; CARBS: 3G; GLYCEMIC LOAD: 2; FIBER: 0G; SODIUM: 389MG; PROTEIN: 11G; FAT: 5G; SATURATED FAT: 0G

Grilled Cauliflower Steaks with Mango and Black Bean Salsa

FERTILITY BOOST, LOWER CALORIE, DAIRY FREE, GLUTEN FREE
SERVES 4 | PREP TIME: 10 MINUTES | COOK TIME: 8 MINUTES

1 large head cauliflower
2 tablespoons extra-virgin olive oil
Salt
Freshly ground black pepper
1½ cups cherry tomatoes
2 cups chopped fresh mango
1 (15-ounce) can black beans, drained and rinsed
¼ cup chopped fresh cilantro
2 green onions, thinly sliced (white and light green parts)
Juice of 2 limes
½ teaspoon ground cumin
1 teaspoon chili powder
½ teaspoon paprika
1 avocado, sliced

1. Remove the outer leaves and extended stem from the head of cauliflower. Working from the center, cut four horizontal, 1-inch-thick steaks. Steaks can only be made with the florets attached to the core stem. Florets that detach from the core can be cooked on the side or reserved for another use.

2. Heat a grill or grill pan to medium-high heat. Brush each side of the cauliflower steaks with some of the olive oil, and sprinkle with salt and pepper. Grill each side for 3 to 4 minutes until lightly charred.

3. For the fresh salsa, cut the cherry tomatoes into quarters and put them in a medium bowl.

4. Add the mango, beans, cilantro, green onions, lime juice, cumin, chili powder, and paprika, and season lightly with salt and pepper. Stir to combine.

5. To serve, place a cauliflower steak on each of 4 plates, and spoon mounds of salsa on top.

6. Garnish with avocado slices and serve.

PER SERVING: CALORIES: 374; CARBS: 56G; GLYCEMIC LOAD: 19; FIBER: 19G; SODIUM: 97MG; PROTEIN: 15G; FAT: 13G; SATURATED FAT: 2G

Kung Pao Tempeh

LOWER CALORIE, INFLAMMATION FIGHTER, DAIRY FREE, GLUTEN FREE
SERVES 4 | PREP TIME: 20 MINUTES, PLUS 10 MINUTES TO MARINATE | COOK TIME: 10 MINUTES

- 8 ounces organic tempeh
- ½ cup tamari sauce
- 1 teaspoon peeled and grated fresh ginger
- 2 teaspoons agave nectar or honey
- 1 garlic cloves, minced
- 1 tablespoon rice vinegar
- 1 teaspoon toasted sesame oil
- 1 tablespoon olive oil
- 1 teaspoon arrowroot powder or cornstarch
- 3 green onions, sliced (white and light green parts), and some for garnish (optional)
- 1 cup snow peas
- 1 medium red bell pepper, chopped
- 1 medium green bell pepper, chopped
- 1 medium yellow summer squash, chopped
- 1 teaspoon crushed red pepper flakes
- ¼ cup unsalted peanuts

1. Set a small steamer basket in a small saucepan over medium-high heat. Add about 1 inch of water and bring it to a boil.

2. Cut the tempeh into 4 slices and transfer to the steamer basket. Cover and steam for about 10 minutes.

3. Meanwhile, in a medium bowl, whisk together the tamari, ginger, agave nectar, garlic, rice vinegar, and sesame oil.

4. Remove the tempeh from the steamer, cut it into bite-size chunks, and add it to the tamari mixture. Marinate the tempeh for at least 10 minutes at room temperature.

5. Heat the olive oil in a large skillet or wok over medium heat. Add the tempeh and sauté gently until it turns golden brown, about 5 minutes.

6. Whisk the arrowroot into the remaining marinade and add it to the pan, stirring the sauce. Add the green onions, snow peas, red bell pepper, green bell pepper, summer squash, red pepper flakes, and peanuts. Cook until vegetables are tender, about 5 minutes, sautéing quickly but gently so the tempeh doesn't crumble.

7. Remove the pan from the heat and serve immediately. Ganish with the remaining chopped green onion (if using).

PER SERVING: CALORIES: 281; CARBS: 22G; GLYCEMIC LOAD: 11; FIBER: 3G; SODIUM: 2023MG; PROTEIN: 18G; FAT: 15G; SATURATED FAT: 3G

Zucchini Pasta with Tomatoes and Peas

LOWER CALORIE, DAIRY FREE, GLUTEN FREE

SERVES 4 | PREP TIME: 10 MINUTES | COOK TIME: 10 MINUTES

- 3 medium zucchini
- ½ tablespoon extra-virgin olive oil
- 3 garlic cloves, minced
- 4 Roma tomatoes, quartered, with their juices
- 1 cup frozen green peas
- Salt
- Freshly ground black pepper
- 2 tablespoons sunflower seeds
- 1 bunch fresh dill, for garnish
- 1 lemon, cut into wedges for serving

1. Feed the zucchini through a vegetable spiralizer or mandoline, or cut it into thin strips with a vegetable peeler.

2. Heat the olive oil in a large skillet over medium heat. Add the garlic and sauté until the garlic is fragrant, 2 to 3 minutes. Add the tomatoes, their juices, and the peas, and cook until the peas are thawed.

3. Add the zucchini pasta to the vegetable mixture. Toss to combine, and cook until the zucchini is heated through, about 3 minutes. Season with salt and pepper to taste.

4. Serve hot, garnished with the sunflower seeds, fresh dill, and lemon wedges.

PER SERVING: CALORIES: 80; CARBS: 9G; GLYCEMIC LOAD: 3; FIBER: 3G; SODIUM: 64MG; PROTEIN: 3G; FAT: 4G; SATURATED FAT: 0G

Vegan "Crab" Cakes

FERTILITY BOOST, LOWER CALORIE, INFLAMMATION FIGHTER, DAIRY FREE, GLUTEN FREE
SERVES 6 | PREP TIME: 20 MINUTES, PLUS 15 MINUTES TO FREEZE | COOK TIME: 8 MINUTES

FOR THE SAUCE

¼ cup mashed avocado

1 tablespoon tahini (sesame paste)

1 tablespoon extra-virgin olive oil

1 tablespoon freshly squeezed lemon juice

Salt

FOR THE "CRAB" CAKES

1 (14-ounce) can hearts of palm, drained and diced

¼ cup mashed avocado

¼ cup diced red bell pepper

¼ cup diced red onion

2 garlic cloves, minced

2 teaspoons Old Bay seasoning

½ teaspoon ground ginger

1 cup cooked quinoa

Salt

Freshly ground black pepper

¼ cup gluten-free flour (chickpea, quinoa, or almond)

2 tablespoons olive oil

TO MAKE THE SAUCE

In a blender, combine the avocado, tahini, olive oil, and lemon juice, and season with salt. Blend until smooth, then pour the sauce into a small bowl for serving.

TO MAKE THE "CRAB" CAKES

1. In a medium bowl, combine the hearts of palm, avocado, red bell pepper, onion, garlic, Old Bay, ginger, and cooked quinoa, and season with salt and pepper. Mix well. Add the gluten-free flour and mix until combined.

2. Form the mixture into 6 rounded patties. Freeze for 15 to 20 minutes (freezing helps them stay together when cooked).

3. In a medium skillet over medium heat, warm the olive oil. Panfry the patties until they are browned on each side, about 4 minutes per side.

4. Serve immediately, passing the sauce at the table.

PER SERVING: CALORIES: 199; CARBS: 20G; GLYCEMIC LOAD: 7; FIBER: 9G; SODIUM: 243MG; PROTEIN: 5G; FAT: 12G; SATURATED FAT: 2G

Split Pea Falafel

FERTILITY BOOST, LOWER CALORIE, INFLAMMATION FIGHTER, DAIRY FREE, GLUTEN FREE
SERVES 4 | PREP TIME: 15 MINUTES | COOK TIME: 50 MINUTES

- ½ cup dried green split peas
- 2 cups water
- ⅓ cup chopped red onion
- 4 garlic cloves
- ½ cup packed fresh flat-leaf parsley
- ½ teaspoon salt
- 1 teaspoon ground cumin
- 1 teaspoon ground coriander
- ½ teaspoon freshly ground black pepper
- 2 teaspoons olive oil, plus more for your hands and for brushing
- 1 to 2 tablespoons chickpea flour
- 2 tablespoons sesame seeds (optional)
- 2 tablespoons tahini (sesame paste) (optional)

1. Preheat the oven to 400°F.

2. In a colander, pick over and wash the split peas. Drain.

3. In a medium saucepan over medium-high heat, combine the split peas and the water. Bring the water to a boil and cook until the peas are tender, 18 to 20 minutes. Drain the peas and let them cool slightly.

4. Put the peas in a food processor (or blender). Add the onion, garlic, parsley, salt, cumin, coriander, pepper, and olive oil; pulse to make a coarse mixture. Transfer to a medium bowl. Add the chickpea flour and stir, as needed, to make the dough less sticky.

5. Line a baking sheet with parchment paper.

6. Grease your hands with some olive oil and shape the dough into 1½-inch balls. Place the balls on the prepared pan. Brush more olive oil on top. Sprinkle with sesame seeds (if using).

7. Bake for 30 minutes or until the falafel is golden and crisp on the outside.

8. Remove the baking sheet from the oven and serve the falafel immediately, with tahini (if using).

PER SERVING: CALORIES: 127; CARBS: 19G; GLYCEMIC LOAD: 7; FIBER: 7G; SODIUM: 301MG; PROTEIN: 7G; FAT: 3G; SATURATED FAT: 0G

Braised Coconut Spinach and Chickpeas

INFLAMMATION FIGHTER, DAIRY FREE, GLUTEN FREE
SERVES 4 | PREP TIME: 10 MINUTES | COOK TIME: 25 MINUTES

- **2 teaspoons olive oil**
- **1 small yellow onion, diced**
- **1 medium red bell pepper, chopped**
- **4 garlic cloves, minced**
- **1 tablespoon peeled and grated fresh ginger**
- **½ cup sun-dried tomatoes, chopped**
- **Zest and juice of 1 large lemon**
- **1 (15-ounce) can chickpeas (garbanzo beans), drained and rinsed**
- **10 gently packed cups baby spinach**
- **1 (14-ounce) can light coconut milk**
- **½ teaspoon salt**
- **1 teaspoon ground ginger**
- **2 large cooked sweet potatoes cut in half, for serving (optional)**
- **½ cup chopped cilantro leaves, for garnish**

1. Heat the olive oil in a large Dutch oven over medium-high heat. Add the onion and bell pepper and sauté for about 5 minutes, or until the onion is beginning to brown.

2. Add the garlic, ginger, sun-dried tomatoes, and lemon zest. Sauté for 3 minutes.

3. Add the chickpeas and sauté for 2 to 3 minutes, or until the chickpeas begin to turn golden and are coated with the onion and garlic mixture.

4. Add the spinach, a handful at a time, and stir. (This will take about 5 minutes. Stir in a handful and wait for it to wilt down and make room in the pot before adding the next handful. Repeat until all the spinach is wilted.) Pour in the coconut milk, salt, ground ginger, and lemon juice. Bring to a simmer, then turn down the heat to low and cook for 10 minutes, or until the chickpeas are warmed through. Taste and add more salt if necessary.

5. Serve over the sweet potatoes (if using) and garnish with the fresh cilantro.

PER SERVING: CALORIES: 405; CARBS: 41G; GLYCEMIC LOAD: 16; FIBER: 11G; SODIUM: 516MG; PROTEIN: 14G; FAT: 23G; SATURATED FAT: 17G

Tofu Kale Scramble

INFLAMMATION FIGHTER, DAIRY FREE, GLUTEN FREE
SERVES 4 | PREP TIME: 5 MINUTES | COOK TIME: 15 MINUTES

- **1 (15-ounce) package non-GMO extra-firm tofu**
- **2 teaspoons olive oil**
- **¼ cup nutritional yeast**
- **1 teaspoon ground turmeric**
- **1 teaspoon paprika**
- **1 teaspoon garlic powder**
- **2 cups stemmed and chopped kale**
- **½ cup halved cherry tomatoes**
- **¼ cup chopped green onions (white and light green parts)**
- **1 large avocado, diced**
- **Salt**
- **Freshly ground black pepper**

1. Drain the liquid from the tofu container, put the tofu block on a plate, and cut it into long strips. Stack the strips on the plate, separating them with paper towels. Place something with a bit of weight (like a heavy dish) on top of the stacked tofu, and set it aside for a few minutes to drain.

2. When the tofu has drained, heat the olive oil in a large skillet over medium heat. Add the tofu strips and use a spatula to break them up into smaller pieces.

3. In a small bowl, stir together the nutritional yeast, turmeric, paprika, and garlic powder. Sprinkle this mixture over the tofu and stir well, so each piece of tofu is seasoned.

4. Add the kale, tomatoes, and green onions to the skillet and cook, tossing frequently, until the kale is tender, about 10 minutes.

5. Stir in the avocado and season with salt and pepper.

6. Serve hot.

PER SERVING: CALORIES: 207; CARBS: 14G; GLYCEMIC LOAD: 5; FIBER: 7G; SODIUM: 113MG; PROTEIN: 14G; FAT: 13G; SATURATED FAT: 2G

Navy Bean and Quinoa Loaf

FERTILITY BOOST, LOWER CALORIE, INFLAMMATION FIGHTER, DAIRY FREE, GLUTEN FREE
SERVES 8 | PREP TIME: 15 MINUTES, PLUS 15 MINUTES TO CHILL | COOK TIME: 70 MINUTES

- **Olive oil cooking spray**
- **3 tablespoons chia seeds**
- **½ cup warm water**
- **1 tablespoon olive oil**
- **1 medium onion, chopped**
- **4 garlic cloves, minced**
- **2 celery stalks, chopped**
- **8 ounces button mushrooms, sliced**
- **1 (15-ounce) can navy beans, drained and rinsed**
- **¾ cup old-fashioned rolled oats**
- **2 tablespoons Bragg's liquid aminos**
- **2 cups cooked quinoa**
- **10 sun-dried tomatoes packed in oil, drained and chopped**
- **1 tablespoon minced fresh thyme**
- **½ teaspoon salt**
- **½ teaspoon freshly ground black pepper**

1. Preheat the oven to 350°F. Lightly coat an 8-by-4-inch loaf pan with olive oil cooking spray.

2. In a small bowl, mix the chia seeds with the warm water and stir well. Refrigerate for at least 15 minutes, until the mixture forms a gel or a "chia egg."

3. Heat the olive oil in a medium skillet over medium heat. Add the onion, garlic, celery, and mushrooms, and sauté for 4 to 5 minutes.

4. In a food processor (or blender), combine the beans, oats, and aminos; pulse until almost smooth.

5. In a large bowl, combine the quinoa, bean mixture, onion mixture, sun-dried tomatoes, chia egg, thyme, salt, and pepper.

6. Transfer the mixture to the prepared loaf pan, pressing it gently to fill the pan and mounding it slightly in the middle.

7. Bake until golden brown and firm, about 1 hour.

8. Remove the loaf from the oven and set it aside to rest for 10 minutes before slicing and serving hot.

PER SERVING: CALORIES: 253; CARBS: 40G; GLYCEMIC LOAD: 16; FIBER: 11G; SODIUM: 421MG; PROTEIN: 15G; FAT: 6G; SATURATED FAT: 1G

Spinach, Sweet Potato, and Lentil Dal

LOWER CALORIE, INFLAMMATION FIGHTER, DAIRY FREE, GLUTEN FREE
SERVES 4 | PREP TIME: 10 MINUTES | COOK TIME: 25 MINUTES

- **1 tablespoon olive oil**
- **1 medium white onion, diced**
- **2 garlic cloves, chopped**
- **1-inch piece fresh ginger, peeled and minced**
- **1 medium sweet potato, diced**
- **1 cup chopped tomatoes**
- **1 small red or yellow bell pepper, chopped**
- **4 cups low-sodium vegetable broth**
- **1 cup dried red lentils**
- **2 tablespoons medium to hot curry powder (or use your own spice mix; see Inflammation Fighter Tip)**
- **2 cups chopped baby spinach leaves**

1. Heat the olive oil in a large skillet over medium heat until it begins to shimmer. Add the onion, garlic, and ginger, and sauté until the onion is translucent, about 5 minutes.

2. Add the sweet potato, tomatoes, bell pepper, broth, and lentils. Cover the pan and simmer for 10 minutes.

3. Add the curry powder (or use your own spice mix) and stir well. Cover and simmer for 10 minutes, until the dal has thickened and the sweet potato is soft.

4. Remove the pan from the heat. Add the spinach, and gently stir until it wilts.

5. Serve immediately.

PER SERVING: CALORIES: 266; CARBS: 45G; GLYCEMIC LOAD: 19; FIBER: 8G; SODIUM: 578MG; PROTEIN: 14G; FAT: 5G; SATURATED FAT: 1G

Baked Broccoli and Bean Burgers

LOWER CALORIE, INFLAMMATION FIGHTER, DAIRY FREE, GLUTEN FREE
SERVES 4 | PREP TIME: 30 MINUTES | COOK TIME: 75 MINUTES

- ⅓ cup uncooked quinoa
- 1 cup water
- 1½ cups broccoli florets
- 2 teaspoons olive oil
- ½ cup chopped green onions (white and light green parts)
- ½ cup chopped red onion
- 2 garlic cloves, minced
- 2 teaspoons ground cumin
- 1 (15-ounce) can chickpeas (garbanzo beans), drained and rinsed
- ¼ cup almond meal or almond flour
- 1 tablespoon tahini (sesame paste)

1. Preheat the oven to 400°F. Line a baking sheet with aluminum foil.

2. Put the quinoa in a fine-mesh sieve and rinse it under cool water, rubbing to remove the bitter outer coating. Drain well.

3. Bring 1 cup of water to a boil in a small saucepan over high heat. Add the quinoa, reduce the heat to medium, and cook for 15 minutes. Drain the quinoa and set it aside.

4. Meanwhile, set a small steamer basket in a small lidded pot and pour in 1 inch of water. Bring the water to a boil over high heat. Place the broccoli in the steamer basket, cover, reduce the heat to medium, and steam for 5 to 7 minutes.

5. Heat the olive oil in a medium skillet over medium heat. Add the green onion, red onion, and garlic, and sauté, stirring occasionally, for 3 to 5 minutes until the onion softens. Remove the skillet from the heat and stir in the cumin.

6. In a food processor (or blender), combine the quinoa, broccoli, onion mixture, chickpeas, almond meal, and tahini; pulse until combined.

7. Form the mixture into 4 patties and place them on the prepared baking sheet.

8. Bake for 50 minutes, turning the patties halfway through. They should be browned and slightly firm to the touch.

9. Remove the patties from the oven and serve hot.

PER SERVING: CALORIES: 299; CARBS: 44G; GLYCEMIC LOAD: 18; FIBER: 11G; SODIUM: 27MG; PROTEIN: 14G; FAT: 9G; SATURATED FAT: 1G

Cauliflower Crust Pizza

FERTILITY BOOST, LOWER CALORIE, INFLAMMATION FIGHTER, DAIRY FREE, GLUTEN FREE

SERVES 2 TO 4 | PREP TIME: 20 MINUTES, PLUS 30 MINUTES CHILLING TIME | COOK TIME: 30 MINUTES

- 2½ tablespoons flaxseed meal or chia seeds (or use 1 whole egg)
- ¼ cup warm water
- ½ medium head cauliflower, chopped into florets
- ⅓ cup chickpea flour (or substitute coconut, almond, or oat flour)
- 1 garlic clove, minced
- ½ teaspoon dried oregano
- ½ teaspoon dried basil
- ½ teaspoon salt
- ½ teaspoon freshly ground black pepper
- 2 tablespoons nutritional yeast (optional)
- ¼ cup chopped fresh basil leaves (optional)

1. In a small bowl, whisk together the flaxseed meal and water, and refrigerate for at least 30 minutes or until thickened.

2. Preheat the oven to 450°F. Line a baking sheet with aluminum foil.

3. Set a small steamer basket in a small saucepan, add 1 inch of water, cover, and bring to a boil over medium heat.

4. Add cauliflower florets to the steamer, cover, and steam until they are soft and falling apart, 3 to 5 minutes. Drain completely.

5. Put the cauliflower in a clean dishcloth or a large piece of cheesecloth, and holding it over a bowl, squeeze out the excess water from the cauliflower. You want it as dry as possible, so at least ⅔ cup water should come out.

6. Discard the cauliflower liquid; the squeezed cauliflower will resemble a firm purée.

7. Place the squeezed cauliflower in a medium bowl and add the thickened flaxseed mixture. Mash and stir well.

8. In a small bowl, mix together the chickpea flour, garlic, oregano, dried basil, salt, black pepper, nutritional yeast (if using), and fresh basil (if using). Mix well. Add the flour mixture to the cauliflower mixture and mix well.

9. Form the dough into a ball and place it on the prepared pan. Pat the dough into a circle and spread it out to a ¼- to ½-inch thickness. You don't want it too thin, because the moisture will cause it to crack.

10. Bake for about 20 minutes, until the top is golden brown and firm to the touch. You can flip it halfway through baking, if you like.

11. Remove the crust from the oven, and reduce the oven temperature to 400°F.

12. Top the pizza crust with your favorite toppings, then return it to the oven and bake for another 8 to 10 minutes or until the toppings have heated. Serve hot.

PER SERVING: CALORIES: 89; CARBS: 8G; GLYCEMIC LOAD: 4; FIBER: 4G; SODIUM: 660MG; PROTEIN: 7G; FAT: 4G; SATURATED FAT: 1G

Fish and Seafood

Grilled Salmon with Pomegranate, Mint, and Pine Nut Couscous

GLUTEN FREE, DAIRY FREE, INFLAMMATION FIGHTER

SERVES 4 | PREP TIME: 10 MINUTES | COOK TIME: 15 MINUTES

- 4 (6-ounce) wild caught salmon filets
- 3 tablespoons extra virgin olive oil
- ½ teaspoon salt
- ½ teaspoon pepper

FOR THE COUSCOUS
- 1 cup dried whole-wheat couscous
- 1 cup water
- 2 tablespoons fresh lemon juice
- 1 tablespoon olive oil
- ½ cup pomegranate seeds
- ½ cup chopped celery
- ¼ cup pine nuts
- ¼ cup fresh mint, chopped plus more for garnish
- ¼ cup fresh parsley, chopped plus more for garnish
- 1 lemon, cut into wedges for garnish
- Salt and black pepper to taste

1. Preheat grill or grill pan. Prepare the salmon by brushing on olive oil. Sprinkle with salt and pepper.

2. Grill the salmon over direct heat on the first side, about 6 to 7 minutes. Turn fish and cook on the second side, about 5 to 6 minutes. Fish should be opaque or reach an internal temperature of 140 degrees.

3. While the salmon cooks, prepare the couscous by bringing the water to boil in a medium pot over high heat. When the water boils, remove pot from the heat, mix in the couscous, cover, and let sit for 5 minutes.

4. Fluff the couscous with a fork.

5. In a large mixing bowl, whisk together olive oil, lemon juice, pomegranate seeds, celery, pine nuts, fresh mint, fresh parsley, and salt and pepper to taste. Add couscous and gently incorporate dressing and couscous with a fork.

6. To serve, divide the couscous between 4 serving plates and top each with a piece of salmon.

PER SERVING: CALORIES: 662; CARBS: 40G; GLYCEMIC LOAD: 24; FIBER: 4G; PROTEIN: 41G; SODIUM: 386MG; FAT: 37G

Salmon, Apple, and Avocado Wrap

INFLAMMATION FIGHTER, DAIRY FREE, GLUTEN FREE
SERVES 4 | PREP TIME: 10 MINUTES | COOK TIME: 15 MINUTES

- **1 pound wild-caught salmon fillet**
- **½ teaspoon salt**
- **¼ teaspoon freshly ground black pepper**
- **2 limes**
- **1 medium tomato, diced**
- **1 large avocado, diced**
- **1 medium apple, diced**
- **1 tablespoon chopped fresh mint**
- **1 tablespoon olive oil**
- **1 head romaine lettuce**

1. Preheat the oven to 425°F.

2. Line a baking sheet with aluminum foil.

3. Place the salmon fillet in the prepared pan. Season with the salt and pepper. Slice one lime and spread the slices evenly on top of the salmon fillet. Bake for 15 minutes, or until the salmon is cooked through. It will look opaque and will flake when pierced with a fork.

4. Meanwhile, in a medium bowl, combine the tomato, avocado, and apple. Set aside.

5. In a small bowl, combine the chopped mint, olive oil, and the juice of one freshly squeezed lime. Whisk to combine.

6. Wash and dry the lettuce leaves.

7. Flake the salmon into the apple-avocado mixture. Add the mint dressing and mix well.

8. Scoop ¼ of the mixture into the center of each piece of lettuce. Roll up to eat.

PER SERVING: CALORIES: 377; CARBS: 19G; GLYCEMIC LOAD: 5; FIBER: 9G; SODIUM: 359MG; PROTEIN: 26G; FAT: 23G; SATURATED FAT: 6G

Fish Tacos

LOWER CALORIE, GLUTEN FREE

SERVES 4 | PREP TIME: 20 MINUTES, PLUS 15 MINUTES TO MARINATE | COOK TIME: 11 MINUTES

FOR THE TACOS
1 pound firm white fish (such as tilapia, cod, or catfish)
2 medium limes, halved
1 garlic clove, minced
1 teaspoon ground cumin
¼ teaspoon chili powder
½ teaspoon oregano
4 teaspoons olive oil, divided, plus more for the grill
Salt
Freshly ground black pepper
½ small head of red cabbage, cored and thinly sliced
½ cup radishes, thinly sliced
½ red onion, thinly sliced
½ cup chopped fresh cilantro
8 (6-inch) organic corn tortillas
Crumbled white cheddar cheese (optional for topping)

FOR THE WHITE SAUCE
½ cup nonfat plain Greek yogurt
1 teaspoon sriracha hot sauce
½ teaspoon crushed oregano
½ teaspoon ground cumin
½ teaspoon dill
Freshly ground black pepper to taste
Fresh lime juice to taste

TO MAKE THE TACOS

1. Place the fish pieces in a baking dish and squeeze a lime half over it. Over the fish, sprinkle the garlic, cumin, chili powder, oregano, and 3 teaspoons of the olive oil. Season with salt and pepper. Turn the fish in the marinade until evenly coated. Refrigerate and let marinate at least 15 minutes.

2. In a medium-sized bowl, combine the radishes, onion, and cilantro and squeeze a lime half over it. Drizzle with the remaining 1 teaspoon olive oil, and season with salt and pepper. Toss to combine, and set aside.

TO MAKE THE WHITE SAUCE

In a small bowl, combine the yogurt, sriracha, oregano, cumin, dill, pepper, and lime juice, and mix until combined. Set aside.

TO ASSEMBLE THE TACOS

1. In a medium skillet over medium-high heat, warm the tortillas one at a time, flipping to warm both sides, about 5 minutes total. Wrap the warm tortillas in a clean dishcloth and set them aside while you prepare the fish.

2. Brush the grates of a grill pan or outdoor grill with oil and heat over medium-high heat until hot. Remove the fish from the marinade and place on the grill.

3. Cook the fish without moving it until the underside has grill marks and is white and opaque on the bottom, about 3 minutes. Flip and grill the other side until white and opaque, 2 to 3 minutes more. Transfer the fish to a plate.

4. Break off some of the cooked fish, place it in a warm tortilla, and top it with the radish mixture, some crumbled white cheddar cheese (if using), and a squeeze of lime. Drizzle with white sauce.

PER SERVING: CALORIES: 290; CARBS: 28G; GLYCEMIC LOAD: 14; FIBER: 3G; SODIUM: 146MG; PROTEIN: 27G; FAT: 8G; SATURATED FAT: 2G

Salmon with Mushrooms and Brussels Sprouts

INFLAMMATION FIGHTER, DAIRY FREE, GLUTEN FREE

SERVES 4 | PREP TIME: 10 MINUTES | COOK TIME: 30 MINUTES

FOR THE VEGETABLES

Olive oil cooking spray

1 pound Brussels sprouts, end trimmed, sliced in half

1 cup shiitake mushrooms

1 tablespoon olive oil

½ teaspoon salt

¼ teaspoon freshly ground black pepper

FOR THE SALMON

1-pound wild-caught salmon fillet, cut into 4 portions

2 teaspoons olive oil

3 garlic cloves, minced

1 tablespoon dried oregano

½ teaspoon salt

½ teaspoon freshly ground black pepper

¼ cup chopped fresh chives, for garnish

TO MAKE THE VEGETABLES

1. Preheat the oven to 450°F.

2. Lightly coat a baking sheet with olive oil cooking spray.

3. In a large mixing bowl, combine the Brussels sprouts, mushrooms, olive oil, salt, and pepper, and toss until well mixed. Transfer to the prepared pan, and spread in a single layer. Bake for 15 minutes, stirring once or twice.

TO MAKE THE SALMON

1. Meanwhile, drizzle salmon portions with the olive oil, and put some of the minced garlic on top of the 4 portions. Sprinkle with the oregano, salt, and pepper.

2. Remove the baking sheet from oven. Move the vegetables over, making 4 empty spots for the salmon fillets. Place the salmon fillets on the pan. Bake the salmon for 10 to 12 minutes until it is cooked through and flakes when pricked with a fork.

3. Let stand for 2 minutes. Serve hot, garnished with the chives.

PER SERVING: CALORIES: 313; CARBS: 13G; GLYCEMIC LOAD: 5; FIBER: 5G; SODIUM: 373MG; PROTEIN: 27G; FAT: 18G; SATURATED FAT: 4G

Thai Halibut and Brown Rice Lettuce Wraps

DAIRY FREE, GLUTEN FREE

SERVES 4 | PREP TIME: 10 MINUTES | COOK TIME: 20 MINUTES

- 4 (1-inch-thick, 4-ounce) fresh halibut fillets
- ¼ teaspoon salt
- ¼ teaspoon freshly ground black pepper
- 1 tablespoon sesame oil
- 2 tablespoons rice vinegar
- 1 tablespoon freshly squeezed lime juice
- 1 teaspoon honey
- ½ teaspoon crushed red pepper flakes
- 1 cup cooked brown rice
- 1 medium red bell pepper, thinly sliced
- 1 cup snow peas, trimmed and thinly sliced diagonally
- ¼ cup thinly sliced green onions (white and light green parts)
- ¼ cup chopped fresh cilantro
- 8 to 12 leaves butter lettuce (Boston or Bibb) or romaine lettuce
- 1 tablespoon cashews, coarsely chopped
- 2 tablespoons chia seeds (optional)

1. Sprinkle the halibut with the salt and pepper.

2. Heat the sesame oil in a large skillet over medium heat. Add the fish and cook for 8 to 12 minutes, or until the fish flakes easily when tested with a fork, turning to brown both sides.

3. In a small bowl, combine the rice vinegar, lime juice, honey, and red pepper flakes.

4. Place one cooked halibut steak on each of 4 dinner plates. Portion out the rice, red bell pepper, snow peas, green onions, cilantro, and 2 to 3 lettuce leaves onto the 4 plates.

5. To eat, spoon some of the fish, rice, vegetables, and cilantro into one of the lettuce leaves. Drizzle with the rice vinegar mixture and sprinkle with the cashews and chia seeds (if using). Roll up to eat.

PER SERVING: CALORIES: 265; CARBS: 18G; GLYCEMIC LOAD: 8; FIBER: 2G; SODIUM: 216MG; PROTEIN: 26G; FAT: 9G; SATURATED FAT: 1G

Asian-Style Haddock in Parchment

LOWER CALORIE, DAIRY FREE, GLUTEN FREE
SERVES 4 | PREP TIME: 10 MINUTES | COOK TIME: 15 MINUTES

- 4 (6-ounce) haddock fillets
- 4 baby bok choy, ends trimmed
- 1 cup small oyster mushrooms
- 1 red bell pepper, thinly sliced
- 1 cup finely shredded green or savoy cabbage
- ½ teaspoon freshly ground black pepper
- 3 green onions, thinly sliced on the diagonal (white and light green parts)
- 2 tablespoons Bragg's liquid aminos
- 1½ teaspoon rice vinegar
- 1½ teaspoon sesame oil
- 2 teaspoons peeled and grated fresh ginger

1. Heat the oven to 400°F.

2. Tear off eight 15-inch squares of parchment paper (you can substitute aluminum foil) and arrange two squares each on two baking sheets.

3. Divide the bok choy, mushrooms, bell pepper, and cabbage evenly among the four parchment squares. Place a haddock fillet on top of each, sprinkle with the black pepper, and top with the green onions.

4. In a small bowl, whisk together the aminos, vinegar, oil, and ginger. Spoon the mixture evenly over the haddock.

5. Top each fillet with one of the remaining squares of parchment, and fold the edges over several times to seal.

6. Bake for 15 minutes or until the fish is easily flaked with a fork.

7. Transfer each packet to a plate. Serve with a knife to split the packet open.

PER SERVING: CALORIES: 194; CARBS: 6G; GLYCEMIC LOAD: 2; FIBER: 2G; SODIUM: 636MG; PROTEIN: 34G; FAT: 3G; SATURATED FAT: 0G

Scallops with Sugar Snap Peas

LOWER CALORIE, INFLAMMATION FIGHTER, DAIRY FREE, GLUTEN FREE
SERVES 4 | PREP TIME: 5 MINUTES | COOK TIME: 10 MINUTES

- 3 teaspoons olive oil, divided
- 12 ounces sugar snap peas, trimmed and sliced diagonally
- 1 medium red bell pepper, sliced
- ¼ teaspoon salt, divided
- ¼ teaspoon freshly ground black pepper, divided
- 2 large shallots, sliced
- 1½ pounds large sea scallops
- 4 lemon wedges

1. In a large skillet over medium-high heat, add 1 teaspoon of the olive oil, and swirl the pan to coat the bottom. Add the snap peas, red bell pepper, ⅛ teaspoon salt, and ⅛ teaspoon pepper, and sauté for 2 minutes. Transfer the snap peas and bell pepper to a bowl.

2. Add the shallots to the skillet and sauté for 1 minute, and then transfer to the bowl with the snap peas and bell peppers.

3. Pat scallops dry with paper towels. Sprinkle evenly with the remaining ⅛ teaspoon salt and ⅛ teaspoon pepper. Add 1 teaspoon of the oil to pan and swirl to coat. Add half of scallops to the pan and cook for 2 minutes. Turn and cook for 1 minute more or until desired doneness. Place the cooked scallops on a plate. Repeat with remaining 1 teaspoon oil and remaining scallops.

4. Serve the scallops with the vegetable mixture and the lemon wedges alongside.

PER SERVING: CALORIES: 223; CARBS: 13G; GLYCEMIC LOAD: 8; FIBER: 3G; SODIUM: 421MG; PROTEIN: 31G; FAT: 5G; SATURATED FAT: 1G

Tilapia and Vegetable Packets

LOWER CALORIE, DAIRY FREE, GLUTEN FREE
SERVES 4 | PREP TIME: 30 MINUTES
COOK TIME: 5 TO 10 MINUTES

- **1 cup cherry or grape tomatoes, quartered**
- **1 cup diced summer squash (like zucchini, yellow squash, or pattypan squash)**
- **1 cup diced eggplant**
- **1 cup thinly sliced red onion**
- **12 green beans, trimmed and cut into 1-inch pieces**
- **2 tablespoons freshly squeezed lemon juice**
- **1 tablespoon extra-virgin olive oil**
- **Small bunch fresh dill, chopped**
- **½ teaspoon salt, divided**
- **1 teaspoon freshly ground black pepper, divided**
- **Olive oil cooking spray**
- **1 pound tilapia fillets, cut into 4 equal portions**

1. Preheat a grill or grill pan to medium heat.

2. In a large bowl, combine the tomatoes, squash, eggplant, onion, green beans, lemon juice, olive oil, dill, ¼ teaspoon salt, and ¼ teaspoon pepper.

3. For each packet, lay two 18- to 20-inch-long sheets of foil on top of each other to create a double layer. Coat the top piece of foil with olive oil cooking spray and lay a tilapia fillet in the center of it. Season to taste with salt and pepper and top with about ¾ cup of the vegetable mixture. Bring the short ends of the foil together, leaving some space in the packet for steam to cook the food. Fold the foil over and pinch it to seal. Pinch the seams together along the sides, making sure they are tight and steam cannot escape. Repeat to make the other 3 packets.

4. Grill the packets until the fish is cooked through and is easily flaked with a fork, and the vegetables are tender, about 5 minutes.

5. To serve, carefully open both ends of the packets, allowing the steam to escape. Use a spatula to place the contents onto plates.

PER SERVING: CALORIES: 174; CARBS: 8G; GLYCEMIC LOAD: 3; FIBER: 3G; SODIUM: 355MG; PROTEIN: 24G; FAT: 5G; SATURATED FAT: 1G

Mediterranean Shrimp Kabobs

LOWER CALORIE, INFLAMMATION FIGHTER, DAIRY FREE, GLUTEN FREE

SERVES 4 | PREP TIME: 20 MINUTES, PLUS 15 MINUTES TO MARINATE | COOK TIME: 8 MINUTES

- 1 pound peeled and deveined jumbo shrimp
- 1 cup cherry tomatoes
- ½ medium red onion, cut in ½-inch cubes
- 12 canned small artichoke hearts
- 1 medium zucchini, cut into rounds
- 1 green bell pepper, cut in 1-inch cubes
- 12 large pitted black olives
- ¼ cup extra-virgin olive oil
- ¼ cup freshly squeezed lemon juice
- 1 teaspoon dried oregano
- 1 teaspoon dried basil
- 1 teaspoon garlic powder
- ¼ teaspoon salt

1. Assemble the skewers by threading the shrimp, tomatoes, onion, artichoke hearts, zucchini, bell pepper, and olives on four 12- to 14-inch skewers in whatever sequence you prefer.

2. In a small bowl, whisk together the olive oil, lemon juice, oregano, basil, garlic powder, and salt.

3. Place the skewers in a shallow baking dish and pour half of the marinade over them; cover and refrigerate for 15 minutes.

4. When you're ready to cook, heat a grill or grill pan to medium heat. Cook the skewers for 3 minutes on each side until the shrimp are opaque and cooked through and the vegetables are soft. Discard the shrimp marinade.

5. Brush the remaining unused marinade on the skewers and cook for 2 more minutes.

6. Remove the skewers from the grill and place them on a serving platter; serve hot.

PER SERVING: CALORIES: 290; CARBS: 11G; GLYCEMIC LOAD: 4; FIBER: 5G; SODIUM: 457MG; PROTEIN: 25G; FAT: 17G; SATURATED FAT: 2G

Halibut with Lentils and Mustard Sauce

INFLAMMATION FIGHTER, DAIRY FREE, GLUTEN FREE
SERVES 4 | PREP TIME: 10 MINUTES | COOK TIME: 35 MINUTES

- 2 tablespoons olive oil, divided
- 1 medium red onion, chopped
- 2 garlic cloves, chopped
- 1 cup Brussels sprouts, halved
- 2½ cups low-sodium vegetable broth, plus ¼ cup
- 1¼ cup dried green lentils, rinsed
- ¾ teaspoon salt, divided
- ¾ teaspoon freshly ground black pepper, divided
- 4 (6-ounce) pieces halibut fillet
- ¼ cup Dijon mustard
- 1 tablespoon chopped fresh tarragon

1. In a large skillet, heat 1 tablespoon of olive oil over medium high heat. Add the onion and cook for 5 to 6 minutes, stirring occasionally, until soft.

2. Add the garlic and Brussels sprouts and cook for 1 minute, stirring occasionally.

3. Add 2½ cups of the broth and the lentils. Simmer, covered, for 20 to 25 minutes, until the lentils are tender. Season with ½ teaspoon of the salt and ½ teaspoon of the pepper.

4. While the lentils simmer, heat the remaining 1 tablespoon of oil in a medium skillet over medium-high heat. Season the fish with the remaining ¼ teaspoon salt and the remaining ¼ teaspoon pepper. Cook 3 to 5 minutes per side, or until opaque and the fish flakes easily with a fork.

5. In a small bowl, whisk together the mustard, the remaining ¼ cup broth, and the tarragon. Divide the lentil mixture and the fish among 4 plates and drizzle with the mustard-tarragon sauce.

PER SERVING: CALORIES: 492; CARBS: 43G; GLYCEMIC LOAD: 20; FIBER: 8G; SODIUM: 646MG; PROTEIN: 52G; FAT: 13G; SATURATED FAT: 2G

Cod with Sugar Snap Peas

LOWER CALORIE, DAIRY FREE, GLUTEN FREE
SERVES 4 | PREP TIME: 10 MINUTES | COOK TIME: 10 MINUTES

- **1 tablespoon freshly squeezed lime juice**
- **1 teaspoon peeled and grated fresh ginger**
- **2 tablespoons olive oil, divided**
- **¾ teaspoon salt, divided**
- **½ teaspoon freshly ground black pepper, divided**
- **4 cups sugar snap peas, strings removed**
- **1 cup button mushrooms**
- **1 medium carrot, peeled and grated**
- **1 tablespoon sesame seeds**
- **4 (6-ounce) pieces cod fillet**
- **1 lime cut into 4 wedges**

1. In a large bowl, combine the lime juice, ginger, 1 tablespoon of the oil, ¼ teaspoon salt, and ¼ teaspoon pepper.

2. Add the snap peas, mushrooms, carrot, and sesame seeds, and toss to coat.

3. Heat the remaining tablespoon of oil in a large nonstick skillet over medium-high heat.

4. Season the cod with ½ teaspoon salt and ¼ teaspoon pepper.

5. Add the fish to the skillet and cook until opaque throughout, 3 to 5 minutes per side.

6. Serve with the vegetable salad and lime wedges.

PER SERVING: CALORIES: 269; CARBS: 10G; GLYCEMIC LOAD: 4; FIBER: 4G; SODIUM: 543MG; PROTEIN: 34G; FAT: 10G; SATURATED FAT: 1G

Poultry and Meat Entrées

Healthy and Easy Chicken Nuggets

LOWER CALORIE, DAIRY FREE, GLUTEN FREE
SERVES 4 | PREP TIME: 10 MINUTES | COOK TIME: 15 MINUTES

- **Olive oil cooking spray**
- **1 pound, boneless skinless chicken breast, cut into bite-size chunks**
- **2 teaspoons olive oil**
- **½ teaspoon salt**
- **½ teaspoon freshly ground black pepper**
- **¼ cup almond flour**
- **1 teaspoon garlic powder**
- **1 teaspoon paprika**

1. Preheat the oven to 425°F.

2. Coat a baking sheet with olive oil cooking spray.

3. Put the chicken in a medium bowl. Add the olive oil and toss to coat the chicken. Season with the salt and pepper and toss once more.

4. In a second medium bowl, whisk together the almond flour, garlic powder, and paprika.

5. Drop a few chicken chunks at a time into the flour mixture to coat, then transfer them to the prepared baking sheet. Repeat with the remaining chicken chunks.

6. Lightly spray the top of the coated chicken chunks with olive oil cooking spray.

7. Bake for 10 minutes. Turn the chicken chunks over and cook for another 4 minutes, or until an instant-read meat thermometer inserted into a larger piece reads 165°F.

8. Remove the chicken nuggets from the oven and serve hot.

PER SERVING: CALORIES: 153; CARBS: 0G; GLYCEMIC LOAD: 0; FIBER: 0G; SODIUM: 364MG; PROTEIN: 26G; FAT: 4G; SATURATED FAT: 1G

Asian Chicken Lettuce Wraps

LOWER CALORIE, DAIRY FREE, GLUTEN FREE
SERVES 4 | PREP TIME: 5 MINUTES | COOK TIME: 15 MINUTES

FOR THE SAUCE
6 tablespoons low-sodium gluten-free soy sauce (or Bragg's liquid aminos)
2 garlic cloves, minced
1 tablespoon honey
2 tablespoons water
1 tablespoon peeled and finely chopped fresh ginger
1 tablespoon rice vinegar
1 tablespoon chili paste
Juice of 2 limes
1 teaspoon arrowroot powder

FOR THE CHICKEN WRAPS
1 tablespoon olive oil
1 pound ground chicken breast
8 green onions, chopped
1 (8-ounce) can water chestnuts, drained, rinsed, and chopped fine
1 red bell pepper, chopped fine
1 medium zucchini, trimmed and chopped fine
1 cup mushrooms, sliced
16 leaves butter lettuce, washed, for wrapping
1 carrot, peeled and grated, for topping (optional)
2 tablespoons finely chopped fresh cilantro, for topping (optional)
2 tablespoons coarsely chopped cashews, for topping (optional)

TO MAKE THE SAUCE

In a small bowl, add the soy sauce, garlic, honey, water, ginger, rice vinegar, chili paste, lime juice, and arrowroot powder, whisk to combine. Set aside.

TO MAKE THE CHICKEN WRAPS

1. In a large skillet, heat the olive oil over medium-high heat. Add the chicken and brown until cooked through, about 8 minutes, sautéing with a wooden spoon and breaking up the pieces. Transfer the chicken to a paper towel–lined plate to drain the fat.

2. In the skillet, add the green onions, water chestnuts, red bell pepper, zucchini, and mushrooms, and sauté for 3 to 5 minutes until soft.

3. Return the chicken to the pan, add the sauce, and cook, stirring, for 2 minutes more.

4. With a slotted spoon, scoop the chicken mixture into the lettuce leaves. Top with the carrot, cilantro, or cashews (if using), and serve hot.

PER SERVING: CALORIES: 351; CARBS: 34G; GLYCEMIC LOAD: 19; FIBER: 2G; SODIUM: 1590MG; PROTEIN: 26G; FAT: 13G; SATURATED FAT: 3G

Quick Pan-Seared Turkey Cutlets

LOW CALORIE, DAIRY FREE, GLUTEN FREE
SERVES 4 | PREP TIME: 5 MINUTES | COOK TIME: 10 MINUTES

- **2 tablespoons olive oil, divided**
- **2 tablespoons freshly squeezed lemon juice**
- **1 teaspoon tarragon**
- **1 teaspoon garlic powder**
- **1 pound turkey cutlets**
- **Salt**
- **Freshly ground black pepper**

1. In a shallow dish, whisk 1 tablespoon of the olive oil, lemon juice, tarragon, and garlic powder.

2. Season the turkey cutlets with salt and pepper, and dredge in the oil-herb mix.

3. Heat the remaining tablespoon of olive oil in a large skillet over medium-high heat. Working in batches, cook cutlets until browned and opaque throughout, 2 to 3 minutes per side. The outside should be nicely browned and the inside fully cooked and opaque, to a meat thermometer reading of 165°F.

4. Let the turkey rest a few minutes before serving.

PER SERVING: CALORIES: 184; CARBS: 0G; GLYCEMIC LOAD: 0; FIBER: 0G; SODIUM: 79MG; PROTEIN: 28G; FAT: 7G; SATURATED FAT: 1G

Walnut-Crusted Pork Tenderloin

LOWER CALORIE, DAIRY FREE, GLUTEN FREE
SERVES 4 | PREP TIME: 10 MINUTES | COOK TIME: 30 MINUTES

- **1 pound pork tenderloin**
- **1 tablespoon mustard powder**
- **1 tablespoon ground sage**
- **1 tablespoon ground rosemary**
- **1 tablespoon paprika**
- **1 tablespoon onion powder**
- **1 tablespoon garlic powder**
- **1 teaspoon salt**
- **1½ teaspoons freshly ground black pepper**
- **½ cup walnuts**

1. Preheat the oven to 375°F.

2. Pat the tenderloin dry with a paper towel.

3. In a small bowl, mix the mustard powder, sage, rosemary, paprika, onion powder, garlic powder, salt, and pepper. Rub the pork tenderloin evenly with the spice mixture.

4. In a food processor (or blender), pulse the walnuts until finely chopped. Coat the pork tenderloin evenly with the chopped walnuts.

5. Place the tenderloin in a baking pan and cook for 30 minutes, or until the internal temperature on a meat thermometer reads 145°F.

6. Let the pork rest for 10 minutes. Cut into slices cross-wise, and serve hot.

PER SERVING: CALORIES: 230; CARBS: 2G; GLYCEMIC LOAD: 0; FIBER: 1G; SODIUM: 640MG; PROTEIN: 25G; FAT: 13G; SATURATED FAT: 2G

Italian Baked Pork Chops with Fennel and Green Beans

INFLAMMATION FIGHTER, DAIRY FREE, GLUTEN FREE

SERVES 4 | PREP TIME: 5 MINUTES | COOK TIME: 30 MINUTES

4 tablespoons olive oil, divided
3 tablespoons freshly squeezed lemon juice
2 tablespoons chopped fresh basil
1 teaspoon ground oregano
4 garlic cloves, chopped
Salt
Freshly ground black pepper
4 bone-in pork loin chops, ½ inch thick
1 fennel bulb, cut into 8 pieces (see Cooking Tip)
3 cups trimmed greens beans
3 jarred roasted red bell peppers, drained and coarsely chopped

1. Preheat the oven to 475°F.

2. In a large bowl, mix 2 tablespoons of the olive oil, the lemon juice, basil, oregano, and garlic, and season with salt and black pepper. Add the pork chops and turn to coat.

3. On a large baking sheet, toss the fennel bulb, green beans, and red bell peppers with the remaining 2 tablespoons olive oil, and season with salt and black pepper. Spread in an even layer.

4. Nestle the pork chops among the vegetables. Roast for 30 minutes, turning the pork chops once halfway through the cooking time, until the vegetables are tender and the pork chops are cooked through, or to an internal temperature of 145°F.

5. Serve hot.

PER SERVING: CALORIES: 330; CARBS: 17G; GLYCEMIC LOAD: 6; FIBER: 7G; SODIUM: 98MG; PROTEIN: 26G; FAT: 18G; SATURATED FAT: 3G

Rosemary and Almond-Crusted Baked Chicken

INFLAMMATION FIGHTER, DAIRY FREE, GLUTEN FREE
SERVES 4 | PREP TIME: 10 MINUTES | COOK TIME: 40 MINUTES

- **1 pound boneless, skinless chicken breasts**
- Salt
- Freshly ground black pepper
- **1 cup raw almonds**
- **4 sprigs fresh rosemary, stemmed**
- **1 tablespoon olive oil**
- **1 medium shallot, minced**
- **2 garlic cloves, minced**
- **2 eggs**

1. Place the oven rack in the middle of the oven and preheat to 400°F. Line a baking sheet with parchment paper.

2. Season the chicken breasts with salt and pepper to taste on both sides. Set aside.

3. In a food processor (or blender), grind the almonds and rosemary until the mixture resembles coarse crumbs. Transfer to a plate.

4. Heat the olive oil in a medium skillet over medium heat. Add the shallot and garlic and sauté until soft, 2 to 3 minutes. Add the rosemary-almond mixture and cook, stirring frequently, until golden brown, 5 to 10 minutes. Transfer to a small, shallow bowl.

5. In another small, shallow bowl, beat the eggs, dredge the chicken in the egg, then dredge it in the rosemary-almond mixture. Press the crumbs to adhere to the chicken.

6. Bake for about 25 minutes, until golden brown, cooked through, and the internal temperature is 165°F. Serve warm.

PER SERVING: CALORIES: 403; CARBS: 8G; GLYCEMIC LOAD: 1; FIBER: 4G; SODIUM: 143MG; PROTEIN: 37G; FAT: 26G; SATURATED FAT: 3G

Chicken Enchilada–Stuffed Spaghetti Squash

FERTILITY BOOST, INFLAMMATION FIGHTER, DAIRY FREE, GLUTEN FREE
SERVES 4 | PREP TIME: 15 MINUTES | COOK TIME: 60 MINUTES

2 small spaghetti squashes
2 tablespoons olive oil, divided
½ pound ground chicken breast
1 cup diced white onion
3 garlic cloves, minced
1 red bell pepper, finely chopped
1 cup cooked black beans, drained and rinsed
1 tablespoon cumin powder
1 tablespoon chili powder
1 tablespoon ground coriander
1 teaspoon salt
1 (8-ounce) can tomato sauce
¼ cup chopped fresh cilantro
1 chopped avocado, for topping (optional)

1. Preheat the oven to 425°F. Line a baking sheet with aluminum foil.

2. Cut the spaghetti squashes in half lengthwise and scrape out the seeds. Place the squash cut-side down in the prepared pan. Bake for 40 minutes or until the squash is easily pierced with the tip of a sharp knife. Remove the baking sheet from the oven and transfer the squash to a cooling rack.

3. Heat 1 tablespoon of the oil in a large skillet over medium-high heat. Add the chicken and brown until cooked through, about 8 minutes, stirring with a wooden spoon and breaking up the pieces. Transfer the cooked chicken to a paper towel–lined plate to drain.

4. Heat the remaining tablespoon of olive oil in the same skillet, add the onion, and sauté for 3 minutes. Add the garlic, reduce the heat to medium, and sauté for 3 minutes, until the garlic becomes fragrant and golden. Turn down the heat to medium low, add the bell pepper, and cook, stirring occasionally, for 5 minutes. Add the beans, chicken, cumin, chili powder, coriander, salt, and tomato sauce, and bring the mixture to a simmer. Turn off the heat and stir in the cilantro.

5. Using a fork, scrape and fluff the flesh of the squash, loosening it from the sides. Evenly divide the meat-vegetable mixture among the 4 halves, mounding it in the center.

6. Return the stuffed squashes to the oven and bake for 10 minutes more, until heated through.

7. Serve sprinkled with some cilantro and chopped avocado (if using).

PER SERVING: CALORIES: 311; CARBS: 35G; GLYCEMIC LOAD: 12; FIBER: 6G; SODIUM: 660MG; PROTEIN: 16G; FAT: 13G; SATURATED FAT: 3G

Grilled Chicken and Avocado Salad

INFLAMMATION FIGHTER, GLUTEN FREE

SERVES 4 | PREP TIME: 5 MINUTES, PLUS 20 MINUTES TO MARINATE | COOK TIME: 10 MINUTES

FOR THE MARINADE

2 tablespoons plain nonfat Greek yogurt
2 tablespoons olive oil, divided
Juice of ½ lemon
4 garlic cloves, minced
1 teaspoon paprika
Salt
Freshly ground black pepper
1 pound boneless skinless chicken breast

FOR THE DRESSING

½ cup plain nonfat Greek yogurt
2 tablespoons red wine vinegar
1 tablespoon olive oil
1 garlic clove, minced

FOR THE SALAD

1 head butter lettuce, washed and torn
1 large avocado, pitted and cubed
½ red onion, thinly sliced
1 cup cherry tomatoes, halved
2 Persian cucumbers, thinly sliced

TO MAKE THE MARINADE

1. In a medium bowl, mix all the marinade ingredients together.

2. Add the chicken, turning to coat on both sides. Cover and refrigerate for 20 minutes.

3. When the chicken is done marinating, heat 1 tablespoon of the olive oil in a large skillet over high heat. Place the marinated chicken in the skillet. Cook the chicken for about 5 minutes per side, to an internal temperature of 165°F. Remove the skillet from the heat.

TO MAKE THE DRESSING

Whisk together the dressing ingredients in a small bowl.

TO MAKE THE SALAD

1. Arrange the lettuce in 4 serving bowls and top with avocado, red onion, cherry tomatoes, and cucumber (if using).

2. Cut the chicken across the grain into thin slices. Divide among the 4 salads.

3. Pour the dressing over the 4 salads and season with salt and pepper.

PER SERVING: CALORIES: 357; CARBS: 15G; GLYCEMIC LOAD: 6; FIBER: 6G; SODIUM: 152MG; PROTEIN: 31G; FAT: 20G; SATURATED FAT: 4G

Herb-Roasted Turkey Breast

LOWER CALORIE, INFLAMMATION FIGHTER, DAIRY FREE, GLUTEN FREE
SERVES 4 | PREP TIME: 5 MINUTES | COOK TIME: 40 MINUTES

- **Olive oil cooking spray**
- **1 pound boneless skinless turkey breast,**
- **1 tablespoon olive oil**
- **2 teaspoons freshly squeezed lemon juice**
- **½ teaspoon freshly ground black pepper**
- **¼ teaspoon salt**
- **3 garlic cloves, minced into a paste**
- **1 teaspoon chopped fresh thyme**
- **1 teaspoon chopped fresh sage**
- **1 teaspoon chopped fresh rosemary**
- **1 teaspoon chopped fresh flat-leaf parsley**
- **⅓ cup water**

1. Preheat the oven to 350°F. Coat a 9-by-13-inch baking dish with olive oil cooking spray.

2. Lay the turkey breast in the prepared pan and lightly spray both sides with olive oil.

3. In a small bowl, combine the olive oil, lemon juice, pepper, salt, garlic, thyme, sage, rosemary, and parsley and stir well to mix thoroughly. Rub the mixture into both sides of the turkey breast. Coat the top with olive oil cooking spray.

4. Carefully pour the water in the bottom of the baking dish to keep the turkey moist. Cover with foil and bake for 30 to 40 minutes or until an instant-read meat thermometer registers 165°F degrees when inserted into the thickest part of a turkey breast.

5. Remove the turkey from the oven and place the baking dish on a wire rack to rest for 10 minutes, keeping it covered with foil.

6. Slice the turkey and serve hot.

PER SERVING: CALORIES: 158; CARBS: 1G; GLYCEMIC LOAD: 0; FIBER: 0G; SODIUM: 201MG; PROTEIN: 28G; FAT: 4G; SATURATED FAT: 1G

Slow Cooker Turkey Breast with Rosemary and Garlic

LOWER CALORIE, INFLAMMATION FIGHTER, DAIRY FREE, GLUTEN FREE

SERVES 4 | PREP TIME: 10 MINUTES | COOK TIME: 4 TO 6 HOURS ON HIGH, OR 7 TO 10 HOURS ON LOW

- Olive oil cooking spray
- 1 cup chopped white onion
- 1 cup sliced carrots
- 1 cup halved Brussels sprouts
- 1 tablespoon minced garlic
- 1 teaspoon chopped fresh rosemary
- 1 teaspoon chopped fresh sage
- 1 teaspoon chopped fresh flat-leaf parsley
- 1 teaspoon paprika
- 1 tablespoon olive oil
- 1 tablespoon freshly squeezed lemon juice
- Salt
- Freshly ground black pepper
- 2 pounds boneless skinless turkey breast

1. Coat the inside of a slow cooker insert with olive oil cooking spray.

2. In the bottom of the insert, arrange the onion, carrots, Brussels sprouts, and garlic.

3. In a small bowl, mix the garlic, rosemary, sage, parsley, paprika, olive oil, lemon juice, salt, and pepper. Brush the seasoning mixture over the turkey breast.

4. Add the turkey to the slow cooker, placing it on top of the vegetables.

5. Cook on high for 4 to 6 hours or on low for 7 to 10 hours, until the turkey is cooked through. Check the internal temperature with an instant-read meat thermometer to make sure it is 165°F before serving.

6. Remove the turkey from the slow cooker and slice it thinly across the grain. Divide the sliced turkey and slow-cooked vegetables among 4 plates; serve hot.

PER SERVING: CALORIES: 320; CARBS: 9G; GLYCEMIC LOAD: 3; FIBER: 2G; SODIUM: 164MG; PROTEIN: 57G; FAT: 5G; SATURATED FAT: 1G

Chicken and Pepper Fajitas

FERTILITY BOOST, INFLAMMATION FIGHTER, DAIRY FREE, GLUTEN FREE
SERVES 4 | PREP TIME: 15 MINUTES | COOK TIME: 11 MINUTES

FOR THE MARINADE

1 tablespoon olive oil

2 tablespoons freshly squeezed lime juice

1½ teaspoons salt

1½ teaspoons dried oregano

1½ teaspoons ground cumin

1 teaspoon garlic powder

½ teaspoon chili powder

½ teaspoon paprika

½ teaspoon crushed red pepper flakes

FOR THE FAJITAS

1 pound free-range, organic boneless skinless chicken breasts, cut into ¼-inch-thick slices

1 tablespoon olive oil

2 red bell peppers, cut into thin strips

2 yellow or orange bell peppers, cut into thin strips

1 medium white onion, cut in half lengthwise, then sliced into thin half-moons

8 romaine lettuce leaves

2 tablespoons chopped fresh cilantro (optional)

TO MAKE THE MARINADE

In a small bowl, whisk together the olive oil, lime juice, salt, oregano, cumin, garlic powder, chili powder, paprika, and red pepper flakes.

TO MAKE THE FAJITAS

1. Put the chicken slices into a large ziplock bag. Pour the marinade into the bag with the chicken. Seal the bag and set aside.

2. Heat the olive oil in a large skillet over medium-high heat. Add the red and yellow bell peppers and the onion, and sauté until the peppers are tender and the onion is turning translucent, about 4 minutes.

3. Transfer the peppers and onions to a large mixing bowl. Cover with foil to keep them warm.

4. In the same skillet over medium-high heat, sauté the chicken slices for 6 minutes, or until they are no longer pink. Return the bell pepper mixture to the pan and sauté to reheat, about 1 minute.

5. Serve the fajitas over the romaine leaves, and top with the cilantro (if using).

PER SERVING: CALORIES: 233; CARBS: 10G; GLYCEMIC LOAD: 3; FIBER: 3G; SODIUM: 661MG; PROTEIN: 27G; FAT: 9G; SATURATED FAT: 1G

Chicken and White Bean Chili

LOWER CALORIE, INFLAMMATION FIGHTER, DAIRY FREE
SERVES 8 | PREP TIME: 15 MINUTES | COOK TIME: 25 MINUTES

- **1 pound boneless, skinless chicken breast,**
- **4 cups low-sodium chicken broth**
- **2 cups chopped Vidalia onion**
- **1 fresh medium jalapeño pepper, seeded and minced**
- **2 garlic cloves, minced**
- **1 (15-ounce) can cannellini beans, drained and rinsed**
- **1 (4-ounce) can diced jalapeño chiles, with liquid**
- **2 cups kale, stemmed and finely chopped**
- **1 tablespoon ground cumin**
- **1 teaspoon oregano**
- **1 teaspoon salt**
- **1 teaspoon freshly ground black pepper**
- **⅓ cup chopped fresh cilantro**

1. In a large heavy-bottomed soup pot or Dutch oven over medium-high heat, add the chicken and the chicken broth, bring the broth to a simmer, reduce the heat to medium, and cook until the chicken is tender, about 15 minutes.

2. Transfer the chicken to a plate and shred with two forks, then add back to the broth.

3. To the pot, add the onion, fresh jalapeño chile, garlic, beans, canned jalapeño chiles, kale, cumin, oregano, salt, and pepper. Stir well to combine. Turn down the heat to low, and simmer for about 10 minutes, until the vegetables are tender.

4. Serve hot, topped with the cilantro.

PER SERVING: CALORIES: 165; CARBS: 19G; GLYCEMIC LOAD: 8; FIBER: 4G; SODIUM: 746MG; PROTEIN: 19G; FAT: 2G; SATURATED FAT: 0G

Turkey Meatballs over Greens

INFLAMMATION FIGHTER, DAIRY FREE, GLUTEN FREE
SERVES 4 | PREP TIME: 10 MINUTES | COOK TIME: 20 MINUTES

- 1 pound 93% to 97% lean ground turkey
- ¼ cup grated onion
- 1 cup grated zucchini
- ¼ cup flaxseed meal
- 1 egg, beaten
- 2 garlic cloves, minced
- 1 teaspoon salt
- ½ teaspoon freshly ground black pepper
- 2 tablespoons chopped fresh flat-leaf parsley
- 2 tablespoons olive oil, divided
- 2 cups Simple Tomato Sauce or 1 (15-ounce) can tomato sauce
- 2 pounds kale, stemmed and roughly chopped

1. In a large bowl, combine the turkey, onion, zucchini, flaxseed meal, egg, garlic, salt, pepper, and parsley. With your clean hands, mix until thoroughly combined.

2. Roll the meat mixture into 1¼-inch meatballs and put on a plate. You should have 26 to 30 meatballs.

3. Heat 1 tablespoon of the olive oil in a large lidded skillet over medium-high heat. When the oil is hot, add the meatballs and brown for 3 to 4 minutes on each side. You may need to cook the meatballs in batches. Use tongs to gently rotate the meatballs so they brown evenly.

4. Reduce the heat to low, add all the meatballs, add the tomato sauce, and cover the pan. Simmer the meatballs and sauce for 10 minutes, or until the meatballs are cooked through.

5. Meanwhile, heat the remaining tablespoon of olive oil in another large skillet over medium-high heat. Add the kale and gently sauté until wilted and tender, about 5 minutes. Turn off the heat and cover to keep the kale warm until the meatballs are done.

6. Put the greens in a large shallow serving bowl, top with the meatballs and sauce, and serve hot.

PER SERVING: CALORIES: 457; CARBS: 38G; GLYCEMIC LOAD: 15; FIBER: 8G; SODIUM: 819MG; PROTEIN: 32G; FAT: 22G; SATURATED FAT: 4G

Open-Face Turkey Veggie Burgers

DAIRY FREE, GLUTEN FREE

SERVES 6 | PREP TIME: 5 MINUTES | COOK TIME: 15 MINUTES

- **1 pound extra-lean ground turkey**
- **1 cup grated zucchini**
- **½ cup finely chopped mushrooms**
- **2 garlic cloves, minced**
- **2 tablespoons chopped green onions**
- **2 shallots, chopped**
- **Salt**
- **Freshly ground black pepper**
- **2 teaspoons olive oil**
- **6 romaine heart lettuce leaves**
- **1 medium tomato, cut into 6 slices**

1. In a large mixing bowl, combine the turkey, zucchini, mushrooms, garlic, green onions, shallots, and season with salt and pepper. Shape into 6 patties.

2. The patties can be cooked on an outdoor grill, in a skillet, or under the oven broiler. To use a large skillet, put it over medium heat and add the olive oil. Warm the oil till it begins to shimmer. Add the turkey patties and cook for about 6 minutes on each side, or until an instant-read thermometer reads an internal temperature of 165°F.

3. Serve the patties over the romaine leaves topped with a tomato slice.

PER SERVING: CALORIES: 137; CARBS: 2G; GLYCEMIC LOAD: 1; FIBER: 1G; SODIUM: 90MG; PROTEIN: 14G; FAT: 8G; SATURATED FAT: 2G

Stir-Fried Pork and Vegetables

LOWER CALORIE, INFLAMMATION FIGHTER, DAIRY FREE, GLUTEN FREE
SERVES 4 | PREP TIME: 10 MINUTES | COOK TIME: 15 MINUTES

FOR THE PORK
4 (4-ounce) boneless pork loin chops, sliced into 2-inch-long thin strips
2 teaspoons arrowroot powder
1½ tablespoons gluten-free low-sodium soy sauce, or Bragg's liquid aminos

FOR THE SAUCE
1½ tablespoons gluten-free low-sodium soy sauce, or Bragg's liquid aminos
Juice of ½ lime
½ teaspoon honey
1 teaspoon toasted sesame oil
2 teaspoons rice vinegar
2 teaspoons Sriracha sauce

FOR THE STIR-FRY
2 teaspoons olive oil
2 teaspoons peeled and grated fresh ginger
4 garlic cloves, crushed
1 cup snow peas
½ cup shredded purple cabbage
1 cup sliced shiitake mushrooms
1 medium red bell pepper, sliced
1 medium yellow summer squash, sliced
¼ cup sliced green onions, for garnish

TO MAKE THE PORK

Put the pork chops in a medium-size baking dish. In a small bowl, combine the arrowroot and soy sauce. Set aside.

TO MAKE THE SAUCE

In a small bowl, combine the soy sauce, lime juice, honey, sesame oil, vinegar, and Sriracha sauce, whisk to mix well, and set aside.

TO MAKE THE STIR-FRY

1. Heat a large skillet over high heat. Add 1 teaspoon of the oil and the pork and sauté 6 to 7 minutes until browned. Transfer to a plate and set aside.

2. To the skillet, add the remaining 1 teaspoon olive oil, ginger, garlic, snow peas, cabbage, mushrooms, bell pepper, and squash. Reduce the heat to low, and pour the sauce over the vegetables. Sauté for 2 minutes.

3. Return the pork to the pan and sauté to reheat, 2 to 3 minutes.

4. Top with the green onions, and serve hot

PER SERVING: CALORIES: 200; CARBS: 11G; GLYCEMIC LOAD: 6; FIBER: 2G; SODIUM: 879MG; PROTEIN: 27G; FAT: 5G; SATURATED FAT: 2G

Drinks and Desserts

Cucumber, Ginger, and Lime Mocktail

LOWER CALORIE, INFLAMMATION FIGHTER, DAIRY FREE, GLUTEN FREE
SERVES 6 | PREP TIME: 10 MINUTES, PLUS 2 HOURS TO CHILL

- **6 medium cucumbers**
- **2 cups water**
- **1-inch piece fresh ginger, peeled and sliced**
- **½ teaspoon powdered stevia**
- **6 tablespoons freshly squeezed lime juice**

1. Set a large strainer over a large bowl. Line it with several layers of cheesecloth or paper towels.

2. Trim the ends off the cucumbers. Cut 6 slices about ¼ inch thick to use for garnish; set aside on a plate. Peel the remaining cucumbers, halve them lengthwise, and scoop out the seeds. Cut into large pieces and transfer to a food processor (or blender); process until the cucumbers are reduced to pulp, about 2 minutes.

3. Pour the pulp into the prepared strainer and use a silicone spatula to press all the juice from the mixture.

4. In a medium saucepan over medium heat, combine the water, ginger, and stevia. Bring to a simmer and cook, stirring constantly, for about 5 minutes. Remove the pan from the heat; remove and discard the ginger slices. Stir in the lime juice.

5. Remove the strainer from the bowl and discard the cucumber pulp. Stir in the stevia-ginger mixture and set the mixture aside to cool to room temperature. Pour the drink into a large jar or pitcher and refrigerate until completely cooled, at least 2 hours.

6. Serve over ice cubes, garnishing each glass with a slice of cucumber.

PER SERVING: CALORIES: 49; CARBS: 12G; GLYCEMIC LOAD: 3; FIBER: 2G; SODIUM: 6MG; PROTEIN: 2G; FAT: 0G; SATURATED FAT: 0G

Coconut Mango Smoothie

LOWER CALORIE, INFLAMMATION FIGHTER, DAIRY FREE, GLUTEN FREE
SERVES 2 | PREP TIME: 10 MINUTES

- **1 tablespoon chia seeds**
- **½ cup water**
- **1 cup unsweetened almond milk**
- **¼ cup canned light coconut milk**
- **¾ cup nonfat plain Greek yogurt**
- **1 tablespoon coconut flour**
- **1 cup frozen mango**
- **1 to 2 Medjool dates, pitted, soaked, and chopped**
- **½ teaspoon coconut extract (optional)**
- **1 cup ice**

1. Place the chia seeds in a small bowl, cover them with the water, and refrigerate for 5 minutes. The chia seeds will soak up the water and form a gel.

2. Add the chia gel to a blender. Add the almond milk, coconut milk, yogurt, coconut flour, mango, dates, and coconut extract (if using). Add more or less ice to reach your desired consistency; process until smooth.

3. Immediately, pour into two tall glasses and serve.

PER SERVING: CALORIES: 362; CARBS: 47G; GLYCEMIC LOAD: 19; FIBER: 6G; SODIUM: 145MG; PROTEIN: 9G; FAT: 18G; SATURATED FAT: 12G

Chocolate Chip Cookie Dough Bites

DAIRY FREE, GLUTEN FREE
SERVES 18 BITES | PREP TIME: 10 MINUTES

- **12 Medjool dates, pitted**
- **½ cup chopped walnuts**
- **1 tablespoon flaxseed meal**
- **1 tablespoon hemp seeds**
- **Pinch salt**
- **¼ teaspoon ground cinnamon**
- **1½ teaspoons vanilla extract**
- **2 tablespoons mini chocolate chips**

1. In a food processor (or blender), combine the dates, walnuts, flaxseed meal, hemp seeds, salt, cinnamon, and vanilla; pulse until everything is well incorporated.

2. Spoon the batter into a medium bowl and fold in the chocolate chips. Roll the batter into 18 bite-size balls.

3. Store the cookie bites in an airtight container in the refrigerator for up to 4 days.

PER SERVING: CALORIES: 80; CARBS: 14G; GLYCEMIC LOAD: 7; FIBER: 2G; SODIUM: 0MG; PROTEIN: 1G; FAT: 3G; SATURATED FAT: 0G

Fudgy Black Bean Brownies

FERTILITY BOOST, INFLAMMATION FIGHTER, DAIRY FREE, GLUTEN FREE
SERVES 9 | PREP TIME: 5 MINUTES | COOK TIME: 25 MINUTES

Olive oil cooking spray
1 (15-ounce) can black beans, drained and rinsed
2 eggs
1 large cooked red beet, peeled and roughly chopped
½ cup raspberries
¼ cup coconut flour
1 tablespoon coconut oil, melted
¾ cup unsweetened cocoa powder
¼ teaspoon salt
1 teaspoon vanilla extract
1½ teaspoons baking powder

1. Preheat the oven to 350°F.

2. Lightly coat a 9-inch square baking pan with olive oil cooking spray.

3. In a food processor (or blender) bowl, combine the beans, eggs, beet, raspberries, coconut flour, coconut oil, cocoa powder, salt, vanilla, and baking powder. Purée for about 3 minutes, scraping down the sides of the bowl as needed, until smooth.

4. Spread the mixture into the prepared pan. Bake for 20 to 25 minutes or until the top is dry and the edges start to pull away from the sides.

5. Let cool on a rack for 30 minutes before slicing. The brownies will be tender, so remove them gently from the pan. The insides are intended to be moist and fudgy.

PER SERVING: CALORIES: 154; CARBS: 21G; GLYCEMIC LOAD: 7; FIBER: 8G; SODIUM: 159MG; PROTEIN: 8G; FAT: 5G; SATURATED FAT: 3G

Raspberry Almond Smoothie

INFLAMMATION FIGHTER, DAIRY FREE, GLUTEN FREE
SERVES 2 | PREP TIME: 5 MINUTES

- 1 cup unsweetened almond milk
- ¾ cup vanilla soy yogurt (or Greek yogurt)
- 1 frozen banana, sliced
- 1 cup frozen raspberries
- 1 tablespoon natural almond butter
- 2 teaspoons wheat germ
- ½ teaspoon vanilla extract
- 1 cup ice, or as desired

1. In a blender, combine the almond milk, yogurt, banana, raspberries, almond butter, wheat germ, and vanilla. Add more or less ice to reach your desired consistency; process until smooth.

2. Immediately, pour into two tall glasses and serve.

PER SERVING: CALORIES: 331; CARBS: 59G; GLYCEMIC LOAD: 21; FIBER: 8G; SODIUM: 138MG; PROTEIN: 9G; FAT: 8G; SATURATED FAT: 2G

Peaches and Greens Smoothie

FERTILITY BOOST, INFLAMMATION FIGHTER, DAIRY FREE, GLUTEN FREE
SERVES 2 | PREP TIME: 5 MINUTES

- 1½ cups unsweetened almond milk
- ⅓ cup frozen edamame
- ½ cup thawed frozen spinach
- 1 cup frozen peaches
- 1 tablespoon hemp seeds
- 2 teaspoons tahini (sesame paste)
- 1 to 2 Medjool dates, pitted, soaked, and chopped (see Ingredient Tip)
- 1 cup ice, or as desired

1. In a blender, combine the almond milk, edamame, spinach, peaches, hemp seeds, tahini, and dates. Add more or less ice to reach your desired consistency; process until smooth.

2. Immediately, pour into two tall glasses and serve.

PER SERVING: CALORIES: 236; CARBS: 36G; GLYCEMIC LOAD: 14; FIBER: 5G; SODIUM: 118MG; PROTEIN: 8G; FAT: 9G; SATURATED FAT: 1G

Iced Ginger Chai

LOWER CALORIE, INFLAMMATION FIGHTER, DAIRY FREE, GLUTEN FREE
SERVES 8 (4 CUPS CONCENTRATE) | PREP TIME: 5 MINUTES | COOK TIME: 20 MINUTES

- 12 cardamom pods, gently crushed
- 8 whole black peppercorns
- 8 whole cloves
- 4-inch piece fresh ginger, peeled and sliced
- 4 cups water
- 4 cinnamon sticks
- 1 teaspoon powdered stevia
- 2 star anise
- 1 vanilla bean, sliced down the middle
- ⅛ teaspoon ground nutmeg
- 4 black tea bags

1. In a large saucepan over medium-high heat, stir together the cardamom, peppercorns, cloves, ginger, water, cinnamon sticks, stevia, star anise, vanilla bean, and nutmeg. Bring the mixture to a boil, reduce the heat to low, cover, and simmer for 15 minutes. Add the tea bags, cover, remove the pan from the heat, and let the mixture steep for 5 minutes.

2. Set a fine-mesh strainer over a large bowl. Pour the tea mixture through the strainer. Discard the solids and let the concentrated liquid cool to room temperature. Pour the concentrate into glass jars and refrigerate until chilled.

3. To serve, mix equal parts concentrate and cold water or milk to make chai tea. Refrigerate in an airtight container for up to 1 week.

PER SERVING: CALORIES: 3; CARBS: 1G; GLYCEMIC LOAD: 0; FIBER: 0G; SODIUM: 0MG; PROTEIN: 0G; FAT: 0G; SATURATED FAT: 0G

Homemade Quinoa Milk

LOWER CALORIE, DAIRY FREE, GLUTEN FREE
SERVES 4 | PREP TIME: 15 MINUTES

- **1 cup cooked quinoa**
- **3 cups filtered water, divided**
- **3 Medjool dates, pitted, soaked, and chopped**
- **1 teaspoon vanilla extract**
- **Pinch salt**
- **¼ teaspoon ground cinnamon (optional)**

1. In a blender, combine the quinoa and 1 cup of the water; blend on high for 1 to 3 minutes until smooth.

2. Put a large sieve over a large bowl and line it with three layers of cheesecloth. Pour the quinoa milk into the cheesecloth over the bowl. The milk will strain slowly on its own, but you can gently squeeze and massage the bottom of the cheesecloth to speed up the process.

3. Put the strained quinoa milk back into the blender and add more of the water 1 cup at a time, blending the mixture after each addition until it reaches your desired consistency. Add the dates, vanilla, salt, and cinnamon (if using) and blend until smooth.

4. Store the milk in an airtight jar in the refrigerator for up to 3 days.

PER SERVING: CALORIES: 32; CARBS: 4G; GLYCEMIC LOAD: 2; FIBER: 0G; SODIUM: 25MG; PROTEIN: 0G; FAT: 0G; SATURATED FAT: 0G

Five-Minute Vegan Hot Cocoa

LOWER CALORIE, INFLAMMATION FIGHTER, DAIRY FREE, GLUTEN FREE
SERVES 4 | PREP TIME: 1 MINUTE | COOK TIME: 4 MINUTES

- 4 cups unsweetened almond milk
- 4 tablespoons unsweetened cocoa powder
- ½ teaspoon powdered stevia
- ¼ teaspoon ground cinnamon
- ½ teaspoon vanilla extract

1. Pour the almond milk into a large saucepan over medium heat and cook until it is just heated through, whisking often.

2. Add the cocoa powder, stevia, and cinnamon, and whisk vigorously to combine.

3. Continue cooking until the mixture is completely combined and the cocoa reaches the temperature you prefer.

4. Remove the pan from the heat. Taste and adjust the sweetness, if necessary. Stir in the vanilla.

5. Pour the cocoa into 4 mugs and serve immediately.

PER SERVING: CALORIES: 132; CARBS: 18G; GLYCEMIC LOAD: 4; FIBER: 3G; SODIUM: 280MG; PROTEIN: 3G; FAT: 5G; SATURATED FAT: 0G

Blueberry Porridge

INFLAMMATION FIGHTER, DAIRY FREE, GLUTEN FREE
SERVES 6 | PREP TIME: 5 MINUTES | COOK TIME: 20 MINUTES

- **1 cup uncooked millet**
- **1 tablespoon chia seeds**
- **½ cup slivered almonds, divided**
- **1½ cups water**
- **1½ cups unsweetened almond milk, plus more for serving (optional)**
- **1 teaspoon vanilla extract**
- **Pinch salt**
- **1 cup frozen blueberries**
- **1 to 2 teaspoons granulated stevia**

1. Place the millet in a small, dry saucepan over medium-high heat and toast for 2 to 3 minutes, until the color deepens slightly and it starts to smell toasty.

2. Transfer to a food processor (or blender). Add the chia seeds and ¼ cup of the slivered almonds, and pulse several times until the millet cracks and has the texture of whole grain flour.

3. Return the millet-almond mixture to the saucepan, along with the water, almond milk, vanilla, and salt. Reduce the heat to medium and simmer for 15 to 20 minutes, stirring frequently, until the millet softens and becomes creamy. Stir in the remaining ¼ cup slivered almonds.

4. Meanwhile, in a small saucepan, combine the blueberries and stevia. Cook, stirring slowly, until the blueberries defrost, 1 to 2 minutes.

5. Serve the millet porridge topped with the blueberries and additional almond milk (if using).

PER SERVING: CALORIES: 249; CARBS: 35G; GLYCEMIC LOAD: 16; FIBER: 6G; SODIUM: 76MG; PROTEIN: 7G; FAT: 10G; SATURATED FAT: 1G

Cherry Chia Pudding

INFLAMMATION FIGHTER, DAIRY FREE, GLUTEN FREE
SERVES 4 | PREP TIME: 25 MINUTES, PLUS 3 HOURS TO CHILL

- 2½ cups unsweetened almond milk
- 1 cup frozen unsweetened pitted dark cherries, thawed
- ½ teaspoon ground cardamom
- ½ teaspoon ground cinnamon
- 1 teaspoon vanilla extract
- 1 teaspoon powdered stevia
- ½ cup chia seeds
- 1 to 2 tablespoons sliced almonds, for garnish (optional)

1. In a blender, combine the milk, cherries, cardamom, cinnamon, vanilla, and stevia and blend on high until smooth.

2. Place the chia seeds in a medium bowl, pour the cherry mixture over top, and whisk thoroughly to combine. Let the mixture rest for 5 minutes, then stir again. After 10 minutes, stir again. Cover and refrigerate for at least 3 hours or overnight.

3. Before serving, give the pudding another stir, then portion it evenly among 4 cups. Top with the sliced almonds (if using).

PER SERVING: CALORIES: 217; CARBS: 24G; GLYCEMIC LOAD: 3; FIBER: 10G; SODIUM: 181MG; PROTEIN: 6G; FAT: 12G; SATURATED FAT: 1G

Cinnamon Bun Mug Cake

LOWER CALORIE, INFLAMMATION FIGHTER
SERVES 1 | PREP TIME: 5 MINUTES | COOK TIME: 2 MINUTES

1 egg
¼ cup old-fashioned rolled oats
1 tablespoon coconut flour
1 tablespoon flaxseed meal
¼ teaspoon baking powder
¼ teaspoon ground nutmeg
¼ teaspoon vanilla extract
¼ teaspoon powdered stevia
1½ teaspoons ground cinnamon, divided
Olive oil cooking spray
2 tablespoons nonfat vanilla Greek yogurt

1. Whisk the egg in a medium bowl. Add the oats, coconut flour, flaxseed meal, baking powder, nutmeg, vanilla, and stevia, and 1 teaspoon of the cinnamon; stir until well combined.

2. Coat a large coffee mug or ramekin with olive oil cooking spray. Pour the batter into the mug.

3. Microwave for 1 minute and 20 seconds or until the cake has puffed up and is no longer wet on top.

4. Top with the yogurt and sprinkle the remaining ½ teaspoon of cinnamon. The mug may be hot from the microwave, so take care.

PER SERVING: CALORIES: 438; CARBS: 37G; GLYCEMIC LOAD: 17; FIBER: 10G; SODIUM: 101MG; PROTEIN: 17G; FAT: 26G; SATURATED FAT: 16G

Banana "Ice Cream"

LOWER CALORIE, DAIRY FREE, GLUTEN FREE

SERVES 4 | PREP TIME: 5 MINUTES, PLUS AT LEAST 2 HOURS TO FREEZE | PROCESSING TIME: 5 MINUTES

6 to 8 ripe bananas (use 1 to 2 per person)
½ cup unsweetened almond milk
1 teaspoon vanilla extract

OPTIONAL ADDITIONS:
Ground cinnamon, cocoa powder, minced fresh ginger
Optional toppings: fresh berries, sliced nuts, chia seeds

1. Peel the bananas and slice them into coins. Put the bananas in an airtight container and freeze them for at least 2 hours, ideally overnight.

2. In a food processor (or blender), combine the frozen banana slices, almond milk, and vanilla.

3. Blend until smooth and creamy, taking two or three breaks to stir the mixture before blending again.

4. Immediately pour the "ice cream" into bowls and serve.

PER SERVING: CALORIES: 190; CARBS: 47G; GLYCEMIC LOAD: 17; FIBER: 5G; SODIUM: 20MG; PROTEIN: 2G; FAT: 1G; SATURATED FAT: 0G

Baked Apples

LOWER CALORIE, INFLAMMATION FIGHTER, DAIRY FREE, GLUTEN FREE
SERVES 4 | PREP TIME: 5 MINUTES | COOK TIME: 30 MINUTES

- **2 large apples**
- 1 teaspoon coconut oil
- 2 teaspoons powdered stevia
- 2 tablespoons almond meal or almond flour
- 4 tablespoons old-fashioned rolled oats
- 2 tablespoons unsweetened almond milk
- ¼ teaspoon ground cinnamon
- **Pinch ground nutmeg**

1. Preheat the oven to 350°F.

2. Line a small baking pan with parchment paper.

3. Cut the apples in half, and remove and discard the core and seeds with a small paring knife or spoon.

4. In a small bowl, combine coconut oil, stevia, almond meal, oats, almond milk, and cinnamon. Spoon on top of the apple halves and sprinkle with the nutmeg.

5. Put the apples on the prepared pan and bake for 30 minutes.

6. Serve warm.

PER SERVING: CALORIES: 119; CARBS: 22G; GLYCEMIC LOAD: 7; FIBER: 4G; SODIUM: 10MG; PROTEIN: 2G; FAT: 3G; SATURATED FAT: 1G

Peanut Butter Blondies

DAIRY FREE, GLUTEN FREE
SERVES 9 | PREP TIME: 5 MINUTES, PLUS 15 MINUTES COOLING TIME | COOK TIME 20 MINUTES

Olive oil cooking spray
1 (15-ounce) can chickpeas (garbanzo beans), drained and rinsed
½ cup natural peanut butter
¼ cup brown rice syrup, or honey or agave syrup
¼ cup coconut sugar
2 tablespoons unsweetened almond milk
2 teaspoons vanilla extract
Pinch ground cinnamon
½ teaspoon salt
½ teaspoon baking powder
½ teaspoon baking soda

1. Preheat the oven to 350°F.

2. Coat a 9-inch square glass baking pan with olive oil cooking spray and set it aside.

3. In a food processor (or blender), combine the chickpeas, peanut butter, rice syrup, coconut sugar, almond milk, vanilla, cinnamon, salt, baking powder, and soda. Blend until creamy and smooth.

4. Pour the batter into the prepared pan and spread it out evenly.

5. Bake for 20 to 30 minutes, until the edges just pull away from the pan, the top is set, and the top is slightly golden brown.

6. Remove the pan from the oven and let the blondies cool for at least 15 minutes before slicing. Serve warm.

PER SERVING: CALORIES: 195; CARBS: 25G; GLYCEMIC LOAD: 10; FIBER: 4G; SODIUM: 96MG; PROTEIN: 8G; FAT: 8G; SATURATED FAT: 2G

Broths, Sauces, and Dressings

Mushroom Gravy

LOWER CALORIE, INFLAMMATION FIGHTER, DAIRY FREE, GLUTEN FREE
MAKES 2 CUPS | PREP TIME: 10 MINUTES | COOK TIME: 15 MINUTES

- 1 cup low-sodium vegetable broth
- 2 tablespoons Bragg's liquid aminos
- 1 shallot, chopped
- 8 ounces mushrooms, stemmed and sliced
- 2 tablespoons arrowroot powder
- 2 tablespoons nutritional yeast
- 2 tablespoons minced fresh thyme
- 1 tablespoon minced fresh rosemary leaves
- ¼ teaspoon freshly ground black pepper

1. In a small saucepan over medium-high heat, combine the broth and aminos and bring to a simmer. Turn the heat to medium-low. Add the shallot and mushrooms, and simmer gently for 10 minutes, stirring occasionally.

2. In a small bowl, stir the arrowroot powder with just enough water to dissolve.

3. When the broth reaches a steady simmer, slowly whisk in the arrowroot slurry, and stir constantly, until the liquid thickens.

4. Remove the pan from the heat and whisk in the nutritional yeast, thyme, rosemary, and pepper. Serve immediately.

5. Store leftovers in an airtight jar in the refrigerator for up to 3 days.

PER SERVING (¼ CUP): CALORIES: 23; CARBS: 4G; GLYCEMIC LOAD: 2; FIBER: 1G; SODIUM: 322MG; PROTEIN: 2G; FAT: 0G; SATURATED FAT: 0G

Simple Tomato Sauce

LOWER CALORIE, INFLAMMATION FIGHTER, DAIRY FREE, GLUTEN FREE
MAKES ABOUT 2 QUARTS | PREP TIME: 15 MINUTES COOK TIME: 40 MINUTES

- **2 tablespoons olive oil**
- **1 medium onion, finely chopped**
- **4 garlic cloves, minced**
- **1 cup finely chopped celery**
- **1 red bell pepper, finely chopped**
- **10 ounces mushrooms, finely chopped**
- **2 (28-ounce) cans crushed tomatoes with their juice**
- **1 tablespoon chopped fresh basil**
- **½ teaspoon dried oregano**
- **Salt**
- **Freshly ground black pepper**

1. Heat the olive oil in a large saucepan over medium-high heat. Add the onion, garlic, celery, bell pepper, and mushrooms and sauté until the onion is softened, 3 to 4 minutes.

2. Add the tomatoes, basil, and oregano, and season with salt and pepper. Bring the mixture to a simmer, reduce the heat to low, and simmer, stirring occasionally, for 30 to 40 minutes.

3. Serve hot.

4. Store the sauce in airtight containers in the refrigerator for up to 4 days, or in the freezer for up to 3 months.

PER SERVING (½ CUP): CALORIES: 42; CARBS: 6G; GLYCEMIC LOAD: 2; FIBER: 1G; SODIUM: 17MG; PROTEIN: 2G; FAT: 2G; SATURATED FAT: 0G

Hemp Seed Dressing

INFLAMMATION FIGHTER, DAIRY FREE, GLUTEN FREE
MAKES 2 CUPS | PREP TIME: 5 MINUTES, PLUS 2 TO 3 HOURS OF SOAKING TIME

- ¾ cup hemp seeds
- ¾ cup water, plus more if needed
- 2 pitted dates
- 3 garlic cloves, minced
- 1 tablespoon apple cider vinegar
- 2 tablespoons freshly squeezed lemon juice
- 1 teaspoon dill
- Salt
- Freshly ground black pepper

1. Put the hemp seeds in a medium bowl and cover with water. Soak for 2 to 3 hours at room temperature or overnight in the refrigerator.

2. Drain the seeds in a sieve and rinse until the water runs clear.

3. In a blender, put the hemp seeds, the water, dates, garlic, vinegar, and lemon juice and blend until smooth. Pour into a medium bowl.

4. Whisk in the dill and season with salt and pepper.

5. Store the dressing in an airtight container in the refrigerator for up to 4 days.

PER SERVING (2 TABLESPOONS): CALORIES: 40; CARBS: 6G; GLYCEMIC LOAD: 1; FIBER: 0G; SODIUM: 6MG; PROTEIN: 2G; FAT: 2G; SATURATED FAT: 0G

Strawberry Vinaigrette

FERTILITY BOOST, LOWER CALORIE, INFLAMMATION FIGHTER, DAIRY FREE, GLUTEN FREE
MAKES 1⅓ CUPS | PREP TIME: 5 MINUTES

- **2 cups fresh strawberries**
- **2 tablespoons balsamic vinegar**
- **1 tablespoon red wine vinegar**
- **1 tablespoon freshly squeezed lemon juice**
- **1 garlic clove, smashed**
- **¼ teaspoon mustard powder**
- **1 tablespoon olive oil**
- **1 tablespoon honey (optional)**
- **Salt**
- **Freshly ground black pepper**

1. In a blender, combine the strawberries, balsamic vinegar, red wine vinegar, lemon juice, garlic, mustard, olive oil, and honey (if using), and season with salt and pepper. Blend until smooth.

2. Serve immediately or store in an airtight container in the refrigerator for up to 4 days.

PER SERVING (2 TABLESPOONS): CALORIES: 27; CARBS: 3G; GLYCEMIC LOAD: 1; FIBER: 1G; SODIUM: 11MG; PROTEIN: 0G; FAT: 1G; SATURATED FAT: 0G

Vegan Alfredo Sauce

DAIRY FREE, GLUTEN FREE

MAKES ABOUT 2 CUPS | PREP TIME: 5 MINUTES | COOK TIME: 5 MINUTES

- **1 (13.5-ounce) can light coconut milk**
- **½ cup nutritional yeast**
- **¼ cup gently packed chopped fresh basil**
- **2 garlic cloves, minced**
- **1 teaspoon arrowroot powder**
- **Salt**
- **Freshly ground black pepper**

1. In a food processor (or blender), combine the coconut milk, nutritional yeast, basil, and garlic; blend until smooth.

2. Pour into a medium saucepan over medium-high heat. Add the arrowroot and stir constantly until thickened. Season with salt and pepper.

3. Serve hot over vegetable noodles, cooked grains, beans, fish, poultry, or vegetables.

PER SERVING (½ CUP): CALORIES: 212; CARBS: 11G; GLYCEMIC LOAD: 5; FIBER: 4G; SODIUM: 40MG; PROTEIN: 10G; FAT: 17G; SATURATED FAT: 15G

Homemade Vegetable Broth

LOWER CALORIE, DAIRY FREE, GLUTEN FREE
MAKES 8 CUPS | PREP TIME: 10 MINUTES | COOK TIME: 1 HOUR

- **4 medium carrots, peeled and roughly diced**
- **4 celery stalks, roughly diced**
- **2 large onions, roughly diced**
- **4 medium garlic cloves, smashed**
- **2 sprigs fresh flat-leaf parsley**
- **2 sprigs fresh thyme**
- **3 bay leaves**
- **2 teaspoons whole black peppercorns**
- **Salt**

1. Place all the ingredients and 1 gallon water in a large soup pot over high heat. Bring to a boil. Reduce the heat to medium-low and simmer for 45 minutes to 1 hour.

2. Pour the broth through a fine mesh strainer into a large heatproof bowl or pot; discard the solids. Cool.

3. Transfer to airtight containers and refrigerate up to 3 days or in the freezer for up to 3 months. Stir before using if the broth separates.

PER SERVING (1 CUP): CALORIES: 12; CARBS: 3G; GLYCEMIC LOAD: 0; FIBER: 0G; SODIUM: 32MG; PROTEIN: 0G; FAT: 0G; SATURATED FAT: 0G

Dairy-Free Pesto

INFLAMMATION FIGHTER, DAIRY FREE, GLUTEN FREE
MAKES 1 CUP | PREP TIME: 5 MINUTES

- **3 cups gently packed fresh basil**
- **½ cup blanched slivered almonds**
- **Juice of 1 small lemon**
- **2 large garlic cloves, roughly chopped**
- **½ teaspoon salt**
- **¼ cup extra-virgin olive oil, plus more if needed**

1. In a food processor (or blender), combine the basil, almonds, lemon juice, garlic, and salt; process into a coarse meal.

2. Slowly add the olive oil in a steady drizzle as you pulse the processor on and off. Process until a smooth, light paste forms. Add enough oil to keep the pesto moist and spreadable.

3. Store the pesto in an airtight container in the refrigerator for up to 5 days.

PER SERVING (2 TABLESPOONS): CALORIES: 117; CARBS: 3G; GLYCEMIC LOAD: 0; FIBER: 1G; SODIUM: 149MG; PROTEIN: 2G; FAT: 11G; SATURATED FAT: 1G

Blueberry Chia Sauce

INFLAMMATION FIGHTER, DAIRY FREE, GLUTEN FREE
YIELD 3¼ CUPS | PREP TIME: 5 MINUTES | COOK TIME: 10 MINUTES

- 2 cups fresh or frozen blueberries
- ½ to 1 cup water
- 2 tablespoons brown rice syrup, honey, or stevia
- 2 tablespoons chia seeds
- 1 to 2 tablespoons freshly squeezed lemon juice (optional)

1. In a medium saucepan over medium-high heat, combine the berries, ½ cup of the water, and rice syrup, and heat, stirring frequently. When the mixture starts to simmer, reduce the heat to medium-low and let simmer for 5 minutes, while breaking down the berries with a wooden spoon. Leave some intact for texture.

2. Add the chia seeds and let the sauce thicken, stirring constantly, for 2 to 3 minutes. Add a bit more water, if needed, until the desired consistency is reached.

3. Remove the pan from the heat and let the sauce thicken for an additional 2 to 3 minutes.

4. Serve over waffles, pancakes, muffins, or Greek yogurt. Store in an airtight container in the refrigerator for up to 5 days.

PER SERVING (¼ CUP): CALORIES: 33; CARBS: 7G; GLYCEMIC LOAD: 3; FIBER: 1G; SODIUM: 1MG; PROTEIN: 1G; FAT: 1G; SATURATED FAT: 0G

Vegan Queso Sauce

FERTILITY BOOST, LOWER CALORIE, DAIRY FREE, GLUTEN FREE
MAKES ¾ CUP | PREP TIME: 5 MINUTES | COOK TIME: 10 MINUTES

- **1 cup unsweetened almond milk, plus more for thickness if needed**
- **1 tablespoon gluten-free flour, plus more for thickness if needed**
- **1 tablespoon olive oil**
- **8 tablespoons nutritional yeast**
- **2 teaspoons Dijon mustard**
- **1 teaspoon Bragg's liquid aminos**
- **½ teaspoon freshly ground black pepper**
- **¼ teaspoon garlic powder**
- **¼ teaspoon onion powder**
- **Salt**

1. In a medium bowl, whisk together the milk and gluten-free flour until smooth.

2. Heat the olive oil in a medium skillet over medium heat. Add the milk mixture and the nutritional yeast and whisk well. Reduce the heat to medium-low.

3. Add the mustard, aminos, pepper, garlic powder, and onion powder, season with salt, and cook, whisking frequently, until the sauce thickens, about 5 minutes. Add more milk or flour to achieve the thickness you desire, if needed.

4. Store in an airtight container for 5 to 7 days. Reheat in the microwave or on the stove top before using.

PER SERVING (¼ CUP): CALORIES: 132; CARBS: 12G; GLYCEMIC LOAD: 3; FIBER: 6G; SODIUM: 235MG; PROTEIN: 11G; FAT: 6G; SATURATED FAT: 1G

Sesame Ginger Miso Dressing

LOWER CALORIE, INFLAMMATION FIGHTER, DAIRY FREE
MAKES 1½ CUPS | PREP TIME: 5 MINUTES

½ to ¾ cup water
½ cup miso
2 tablespoons rice vinegar
2 tablespoons low-sodium soy sauce
2 tablespoons sesame oil
3 garlic cloves, minced
1 teaspoon peeled and minced fresh ginger
½ teaspoon onion powder

1. In a blender, combine the water, miso, vinegar, soy sauce, sesame oil, garlic, ginger, and onion powder. Blend until smooth.

2. Store the dressing in the refrigerator in an airtight container up to 4 days.

PER SERVING (2 TABLESPOONS): CALORIES: 46; CARBS: 3G; GLYCEMIC LOAD: 2; FIBER: 1G; SODIUM: 595MG; PROTEIN: 2G; FAT: 3G; SATURATED FAT: 0G

Printed in the USA
CPSIA information can be obtained
at www.ICGtesting.com
LVHW070747300124
770336LV00030B/653